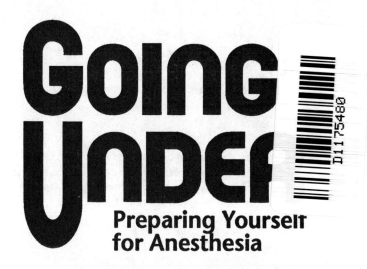

# GOING UNDER

## Preparing Yourself for Anesthesia

**Y**our Guide to Pain Control
and Healing Techniques –
Before, During and After
Surgery

*Monica Winefryde Furlong, M.D.*

*Elliot T. Essman*

Autonomy Publishing Corporation
New York, New York

Published by
Autonomy Publishing Corporation
501 East 87th Street, Suite 15B
New York, NY 10128
(212) 288-0095; Fax: (212) 794-4996


Printed and bound in the United States of America
Cover design by Robert Howard


Library of Congress Catalog Card Number 93-072364


Publisher's Cataloging in Publication
        *(Prepared by Quality Books Inc.)*
Furlong, Monica Winefryde, 1940 —
        Going under : preparing yourself for anesthesia and
        pain control / Monica Winefryde Furlong, Elliot Essman.
        p. cm.
        Includes bibliographical references and index.
        ISBN 0-9636451-6-1

        1. Anesthesia — Popular works. 2. Analgesia — Popular works.
        3. Pain, Postoperative. I. Essman, Elliot T. II. Title

RD81.F87 1993                    617.96
                                 QBI93-995

To surgical patients everywhere...

And to the dedicated doctors and nurses who care for them.

# Disclaimer

*Going Under* is a book designed to inform people without medical training about surgery, anesthesia and postsurgical pain control. It is designed to provide general information, but is not intended to be a substitute for the advice of your own physician or health care provider.

While every effort has been made to make sure that the information provided in *Going Under* is accurate and up to date, the book may contain inaccuracies and typographical errors. As such, it is to be used as a general guide to the subject only. It is not meant to serve as a definitive technical textbook.

One of the premises of this book is that each situation and each patient is unique. Hence, before you or someone you care about goes through anesthesia and surgery, it is important that you consult your physician to obtain information relevant to your own individual case and to have the physician answer any questions you might have about anesthesia and pain control.

Many of the medications and drugs we mention in this book by their generic names are well known to the general public; however, we prefer not to use trade names. Once again, it is important to consult your doctor about the use of any technique, drug or medication.

# Table of Contents

# Preface

➤ You're going in for surgery. Even routine surgery can bring difficulty and uncertainty. So you've covered every angle you can possibly think of, talked to everybody you can find who's had similar surgery, gotten second and even third opinions. But it's not likely that you've given much thought to anesthesia. Most people don't. And yet without anesthesia modern surgery would not be possible. Before your surgeon can operate on you, you need anesthesia to prevent pain. After the operation you may have further pain and will need some help in controlling it too.

Pain will be a major character in this story — the villain, in fact. Pain has henchmen and cronies — worry, fear, anxiety — that help it do its damaging work. But pain is no match for the inner strength of the human being — *your* inner strength, *your* courage, *your* will to live a healthy, fulfilling life.

Pain is more like a petty criminal — easily managed, reformed, and put in its place, once you know the proper techniques.

Pain thrives on ignorance; knowledge drives pain away. Pain breeds on fear; belief in yourself keeps pain in check.

Pain fills the vacuum of our inaction; communicating your needs can banish it.

But *you* have to do something. You can't close your eyes and leave pain control to the doctors. No matter how skilled they are, no matter how caring, they can't feel *your* pain. You're a member of the medical team taking care of you, and you have just as active a part to play in seeing that the operation and your recovery are the very best possible.

During your operation the surgeon, with all the tools of modern technology, gets to see everything. You, on the other hand, see nothing. The anesthesiologist takes care of that. You miss all the excitement. You sleep right through it...

...or do you? More and more, fast breaking research suggests that although you seem to be asleep under anesthesia, your brain may actually be registering certain stimuli. Even if you don't remember, hearing does occur.

The more you know, the more you prepare, and the more you insist on your rights and personal dignity as a patient, the smoother and safer your surgery and recovery will go. Your healing process is *your* affair. *You* are the one who will feel the post-surgical pain.

The purpose of this book is to give you the tools to make pain a small thing when you, or someone you love, must undergo surgery. Whether you browse through sections that catch your eye or read the book cover to cover, you'll learn more about what pain is and what healing is. You'll learn why people are subject to unnecessary pain during and after surgery and what you can do about it. Most important, you'll learn how to direct your mind and body to work together so you'll leave the hospital as healthy as you can possibly be.

# Acknowledgments

We wish to thank the many people who helped and encouraged us to write *Going Under*, particularly the wonderful patients, surgeons, anesthesiologists, nurses and staff of Beth Israel Medical Center North in New York City.

Specifically, we'd like to give our warm thanks to Beth Brodman, MD for her comments on pediatric anesthesia; Michele Chotkowski, RN for the perspective she gave us on the role of the nursing profession; André Clavel, MD for his comments on acupuncture; Nina Ann Essman, JD for her expert proofreading and editing; Michele Fumiere, MD for her clinical work with Dr. Furlong's anesthesia suggestion cassettes; Judy Halevi for her inspiration and expertise in producing our intraoperative suggestion cassette tape; Robert Howard for his excellent book cover design; Sundar Koppolu, MD for his review of the manuscript and comments on anesthesia practice; Rohini Lingham, MD for her review of the manuscript; Peter Meade, MD for his comments on emergency surgery; Diane Moore, RN, Ph.D. for her contributions to the chapter on anesthesia in childbirth; Penelope Otton for her top-notch professional editing of the manuscript; Rosa Razaboni, MD for her support and encouragement; W. Campion Read, MD for his unwavering support, careful reading of the book and trenchant comments; Richard Scuderi, MD for his contributions to the chapter on anesthesia in childbirth; and Jeanette Tracy for her courageous recounting of her experience of awareness while under general anesthesia.

Irwin Lear, MD; Avram Cooperman, MD; Wendy Monkcom, MD; and Jack Rudick, MD have given Dr. Furlong special support and encouragement in her research on awareness under anesthesia and have been strong supporters of this book.

We'd also like to thank Henry L. Bennett, Ph.D.; Jane Brendel; Anthony Cahan, MD; Raymond Douglas Davies; Peggy Huddleston; John F. Kihlstrom, Ph.D.; Jason W. Kwee, MD; Ilkley LaChienne; Morrison S. Levbarg, MD; Bernard Levinson, MD; Laurie Lewis, MD; Ellen Marsh; Michael O'Leary, MD; and Linda Rogers, C.S.W. for their advice, encouragement and general contributions to *Going Under*.

# Introduction

>> Anesthesia is more than just a specialized branch of medicine. It's more than the knowledge of how to prepare a person to go through surgery without feeling pain. It's the art (and it is an art) of guiding you—both in mind and body—through a period in which you're *as helpless as a baby*.

The hospital staff are superbly trained, but they simply don't have time to see your point of view. To them you become the "hysterectomy," the "tonsils," or the "gall bladder." You are vulnerable, you feel powerless, and you don't even have your clothes on to protect you from the elements. You are prey to fear, anxiety, discomfort, and pain. But the worst thing is not knowing what is going to happen. New ground can be difficult for the bravest among us.

Surgery takes enormous trust. We may consider ourselves brave. We might, on the other hand, freely admit that we are scared stiff. We may never have given the matter real thought before the day scheduled for surgery. Yet most of us will approach the surgery/anesthesia process like a child groping in the darkness for help. Good anesthesiologists and the nursing professionals who back them up see their profession in this larger sense. Even for experienced anesthesiologists, giving anesthesia can be stressful. So they know how much more stressful the situation can be for the patient. They realize how helpless and lonely the patient may feel. They realize they have the power to make a real difference toward the patient's recovery.

Surgery spells "c-r-i-s-i-s" for most people — and that's normal. The concerns you have can mount and snowball. Even if the surgery is minor, the very need for surgery may underscore the fact that you are growing older, and feel more fragile, less in control of your body. You are being thrust suddenly into a hospital setting where pain, illness, and even death are commonplace.

Many worries can surface. Will they use the right techniques for controlling pain? Will my body be mutilated or disfigured by the surgery? When they open me up, will they find further evidence of disease and decay? Will it be cancer? Will I react badly to the anesthesia? How quickly will I recover? How soon will I be able to resume my normal life? Will I have open-ended financial liabilities? Can I really trust all these people to do their best? What if something goes very, very wrong?

You're in an unfamiliar setting — the hospital. No matter how fine a hospital, you hear more about illness and pain than about health. That's to be expected. All this can bring uncomfortable feelings out of the woodwork. Even people facing minor surgery may be reluctant to admit how terrified they are. Pain, even in minor surgery, can be severe if not properly managed. The mind, which can deal with pain very well by lessening it, can also make it worse.

Good, sympathetic surgeons or anesthesiologists do their patients a real service by helping them to admit that they are anxious. Says Dr. Campion Read, an anesthesiologist in New York City:

*After you probe a little bit with them, they often do admit that they are frightened. That's the key to working on the fear. Unrecognized fear is the most damaging. And if you sit down with them and probe a little bit, you uncover things: one of their parents died when they were young, or died at the same age they are now. They might discover unpleasant memories of being hospitalized as a child, where they had inadequate preparation and were very fearful, even if it was something many of their friends went through without much trouble — their tonsils or appendix. Once they get in touch with this, it usually helps them get rid of the terror. But still, it's hard to completely erase some people's irrational fears of dying from minor surgery.*

As we shall see, courage and belief in yourself (and your health) is important. But getting information — real learning about the issues and problems you will face — is the first step. The better informed you are about surgery and pain control, the more positive your experience will be. Many new techniques, such as the use of narcotics to specifically target pain receptors, are coming into use. Time-honored mental and emotional methods of dealing with pain and fear are also available. But you as a patient are simply not a wise consumer unless you attain an understanding of what you will be going through.

Your anesthesiologist will know how to make you physically secure and comfortable before, during, and after the surgery. He or she will also try to make you feel more *emotionally* secure. But because your anesthesiologist gets to speak with you for only a short time, you have to do some emotional preparation on your own. You have got to add your *own* efforts toward making the experience a success.

Once you are given general anesthesia and are ready to undergo surgery, the most critical period of all begins. It is a period of total helplessness on your part and absolute trust. Both you and the anesthesiologist hope and expect that you will feel nothing under anesthesia, and that afterwards you will remember nothing. But, as we shall see, it's not that simple. Both psychologists and physicians are conducting research on the critical questions of what patients hear and are aware of during surgery. The possibilities are fascinating. Some anesthesiologists are experimenting with guiding their patients through sophisticated mental preparation techniques. Others are experimenting with audiotaped suggestions played to patients during surgery. It's all in an attempt to make surgery less frightening, to make pain less of a lingering problem, to make recovery all the more rapid.

The resources you can use to make your anesthesia and surgery experience the best possible are out there in abundance. There are many areas to explore, many choices to make. But the key to understanding your choices can be boiled down to a pair of related themes: what you put into your body, what you put into your mind. What ties these two together is the fact that *you* must become active in ensuring the best possible care that you can obtain. *You* must come to understand your own personal physical and emotional needs. *You* must learn what you yourself can do to improve your surgical experience. Hospital patients are not used to taking an active part in their own care. There are things *you* can do, choices *you* can make that will have very positive effects on your surgical outcome and recovery. This book will give you easy-to-learn techniques you can use to get fully involved.

# One

# Body and Mind Together

*Mind moves matter.*

Virgil

>> The mind affects the body. The body affects the mind. It's not always easy – or even useful – to clearly differentiate between the two. In anything we do, the mind – our mental attitudes, fears, weaknesses, and inner strengths – can affect how we react physically. This is true in your work, sports, and your sex life. It is certainly true when we deal with anesthesia, surgery, and recovery.

For example, anesthesiologist Lawrence Egbert conducted an experiment back in the 1960s that dramatically reduced patient pain. He simply instructed his patients to relax the muscles around their surgical incisions. They used less medication; they went home earlier.

We'll be covering many techniques that merge mind and body and that get you back on your feet earlier, with less pain. But one thing ties all the techniques together: you must take an active role. It's your body, your surgery, your pain, your healing, your recovery, your health.

During your hospitalization, you can speak up to make sure you get the best possible professional attention. You can also prepare yourself to make sure that what goes into your body and what goes into your mind, all lead to the best possible surgical experience for you.

Let's be more specific. What actually goes into your body? Mainly drugs. That's right, the *D* word. The primary definition of *drug* in the dictionary is *any substance used as a medicine or as an ingredient in a medicine*. The secondary definition is *a narcotic, hallucinogen, etc., especially one that is habit-forming*. In our everyday thinking, too often we opt for the second definition. We forget how beneficial drugs can be, how they save lives and alleviate pain. Too often when we hear the word *drug*, we follow it by the word *abuse*. The fact that drugs carry such a stigma in our society today is not the subject of this book. But the proper use of drugs is. There are legitimate and proper uses (*abuse* without the *ab*) for narcotic drugs. In a hospital, during and after surgery, to alleviate pain, to hasten recovery, and to maintain personal wholeness — all are legitimate uses in the mainstream of our culture.

Narcotic drugs are necessary both during and after surgery. There is nothing wrong with them. But because of the hysteria about drugs, because of the stigma attached to them, some of the people taking care of you at the hospital may be tempted to deprive you of drugs you need. It's the "just say no" way of thinking, and it is uncalled for. You may suffer both mentally and physically as a result. We'll be examining the problem of undermedication later, in detail.

What goes into your mind. Critical. When you are lying in a hospital bed staring at the ceiling, negativity can take over. Fear can grip you. Stray remarks can agitate you. But your own attitude can guide you through these tough times if you really want it to. What's more, you can also insist on your rights to dignified and proper surroundings before, during, and after surgery. We'll be covering at length the fast-breaking research on consciousness *during* surgery, and how listening to music and suggestion cassettes, even those you prepare yourself, can help improve your healing and recovery.

Mind and body are not merely linked; in reality they are one. While mind and body linkages are a popular subject lately, the idea is nothing new. The ancient Greeks and Romans took the idea as a given. The time-honored traditions of Chinese and Indian medicine have always treated mind and body together as a holistic one.

> For most of human history, mind and body were not thought of separately. Only for the past five hundred years or so, as medicine has become more and more "scientific," has the study of what ails the body diverged from the study of what ails the mind. For us once again to treat mind and body as a holistic unity is to take a major step toward effective health.

But this is no place for theory or history. Let's look at two examples, one positive, one negative, of mind-body connections that affect the question of surgical pain, anesthesia, and healing. That's *your* pain we're talking about.

You, the patient, enter the hospital. You are knowledgeable about pain control, the types of drugs you'll receive. The anesthesiologist explains procedures to you fully. You have the support of friends and family. You have practiced self-hypnosis, visualization, or meditation exercises at home. You arrange to listen to a cassette of music or positive suggestions for healing while you are under anesthesia. The hospital's pain control service works with you closely after surgery. You heal rapidly and leave the hospital earlier than expected. You get back to work more quickly too.

The other extreme. You go into surgery unprepared. You know little or nothing about the procedures you will be going through. Your hospital has no pain management service and you receive an inadequate level of medication. During surgery, you may not feel that you have lost consciousness completely. You may vaguely remember remarks made by surgical personnel while you were supposedly "asleep." When you wake up from anesthesia, you feel negative and uneasy. You suffer needless physical and emotional pain. Your healing takes its sweet time. While the doctors do eventually let you out of the hospital after declaring your surgery a "success," you're still a long way from feeling well. You carry psychic as well as physical scars.

Let's say you wake up after minor surgery feeling uneasy, having bad dreams, even losing your appetite. The reason: the surgeons were discussing pain and cancer — somebody else's — all through your operation. That's not your fault of course, but aware, informed patients would have used music or suggestion cassettes during general anesthesia to shield themselves against damaging mental input of just this sort.

One of the authors, Dr. Furlong, had a well-informed patient who specifically asked that no negative comments be uttered during her surgery. Dr. Furlong passed this request on to the rest of the surgical team. To lighten the atmosphere further, Dr. Furlong felt obliged to single out one of the surgeon's assistants and ask him not to speak at all; *everything* he said was negative.

The key to this book is this: mind and body work together. And it's the key to the best outcome possible of your surgery. You have to help create it—you and the rest of the surgical team together. The mind/body unity we're talking about here is yours; you are you, and not "just a patient." You might receive excellent medical care if you don't speak up, but don't count on it. If you do pay attention, if you become an informed patient, you'll stand the best chance of getting the medications that are right for you — of focussing on the positive. Pain will be something remote, easy to deal with, a detail of your surgery — not the central feature. You will be home and back to normal activities quickly. Healing will be your theme. And the best part of it all is, you helped yourself to get well.

# Two

# Pain

*Pain is no evil unless it conquers us.*
George Eliot

» Pain, as we shall see, is a uniquely personal phenomenon. The pain one person shrugs off can cripple someone else. Any doctor or nurse who works in an emergency room can tell stories of injured people who should be in unbearable pain—but somehow the pain skips them. Your pain is affected by who you are. Your expectations matter. So does what you're thinking about when the pain occurs. Your brain acts as a clearing house for your body's pain. Your brain can magnify your pain, but it can also control and minimize it.

*Just what is pain anyway,* you ask? *I thought I knew until you came along to complicate things.* Pain, distilled, is information. It is an uncomfortable feeling that tells you that somewhere in your body something may be going wrong. Pain is your body's way of sending a warning to your brain. Your nervous system — the nerves and spinal cord — act as a highway for messages to and from your brain and the rest of your body.

Receptor nerve cells in and beneath your skin sense heat, cold, light touch, pressure — and pain. All of us have multitudes of these receptor cells. Some cells are few in number, like the sensors for cold. The pain sensors are the most numerous. When there is an injury to your body, these tiny cells send messages along your nerves into your spinal cord and then up to your brain. And since the earliest days of medical science, in every culture, healers have sought ways to short-circuit these messages, to stop them from reaching the brain.

Pain is not just a physical feeling—it's an emotional feeling. Your physical makeup affects how you feel pain, but so does your psychological makeup. There is even a sociological factor—people from different cultures react to pain differently. Like pleasure, the experience of pain is highly personal.

True, no one else can guess or imagine exactly how you feel pain, not even pain control professionals. But that's not bad news really. Since pain *is* personal, you can get to know it, understand it, and keep it under control.

And you are not alone. As much as you want to do your bit against your own pain, modern medicine wants to help you do it. Pain researchers hope, within twenty years, to have the ability to eliminate pain completely, with total safety. Even now, though pain can't yet be simply "shut off," it can be reduced. It can be managed. The most damaging aspects of pain can be brought under control.

Pain control, in the medical sense, can be divided neatly into two major areas. One area deals with the control of chronic pain or pain related to various diseases, ranging from backaches and headaches to arthritis and advanced cancer. This is not one of medicine's "glamour" areas— but it is important to millions of people.

The second area—our area, anesthesia and post operative pain management—deals with eliminating pain during surgery and managing or controlling pain after surgery.

We take a holistic view of pain. It's the human being, the person, who feels the pain. Not just the mind. Not just the body. But both, together. And we're not talking about scraping your knee at the playground; this is *real surgery*. In the hospital, the emotional stress, fear, and uncertainty you might feel not only increase the pain, they are themselves pain. In taking control of your pain you'll deal with all these issues as a unit.

Don't assume that procedures for handling surgical and postsurgical pain are uniform or standard wherever you go for your surgery. You'll pay for this misconception in physical pain and a slower recovery from surgery. You'll even pay in dollars and cents. Unless you're hit by a truck and rushed to a hospital for emergency surgery, you have the ability to do basic consumer research. Not only can you short-circuit your pain and make healing easier, you can even save money by shortening your hospital stay.

Postsurgical pain is a national issue. In March of 1992, a panel of experts convened by the federal government's Agency for Health Care Policy caused quite a stir. In a news conference jointly sponsored by the Agency and the American Medical Association, they announced some striking findings. On average, the panel said, the dosages of conventional pain medication given after surgery are less than *half* the amount required to control the pain effectively. That means that patients *usually* don't get enough of the pain killer they need.

Why is the practice of giving inadequate pain medication so widespread? The panel reported that patients were often denied the proper level because of certain pervasive medical myths—most notably that morphine and related drugs, even if put to proper medical use, may lead to addiction. Another myth holds that infants and the elderly can withstand a great deal of pain. Yet another myth holds that pain in itself is not harmful; some people even think that it builds character.

Drug addiction is a serious problem, but the panel stressed that addiction is extremely rare when the drugs are used properly. The panel cited a study of twelve thousand patients given opiates (drugs like *morphine*, *meperidine*, *dilaudid* and *methadone*) for acute pain. Fewer than five became drug-tolerant or addicted. The vast majority of patients who receive pain-killing opiates over a long time period never become addicted. And they do get major relief from devastating pain.

> Pain killing drugs, especially narcotics, have a proper place — to control pain for patients during and after surgery. Addiction and other problems usually associated with abuse of narcotics are the stuff of the street, not the recovery room.

Finishing their testimony, the panel strongly urged patients to work closely with their doctors, exploring the full range of options for handling pain. No matter how good the doctors and nurses may be, they cannot personally feel the patient's pain. The doctor must listen to the patient, but the patient also has a responsibility to give the doctor usable information about the pain. The doctor can't do much for the patient if the patient does little more than gripe and complain.

We see how pain has become a national issue. It's a community issue and a hospital issue. Most important, it's *your* personal issue.

Pain is one of the great scourges of the human condition. Without control of pain, your surgery would simply not be possible. To vanquish pain entirely or to bring it down to a bearable level, we turn to the art and science of anesthesia.

# Three

# Types of Anesthesia

*The art of life is the art of avoiding pain.*

Thomas Jefferson

» Medicine and surgery have been practiced in some form or other since the beginning of civilization. Even early Egyptian writings tell of a vast array of surgical procedures performed on nearly every part of the human body. Over 2,000 years ago Indian physicians were able to remove urinary stones. Some of these early practitioners had devised methods for relieving pain during surgery, but until relatively recent times, most pain control methods involved stupefying the patient with substances like alcohol, which are not really effective or consistent pain killers.

Anesthesia as we know it is a comparatively recent phenomenon. Up until the mid-nineteenth century, most medical treatment did not involve surgery. The surgeon might saw off and cauterize an arm or a leg damaged in an accident or a battle, but rarely would the surgeon dare to enter a body space such as the abdomen or a joint. Infection was a major problem, of course, but surgical pain was an even greater problem. Without effective techniques for controlling pain, the surgeon could not afford to spend more than a few minutes working on the patient. So surgeons had to work fast. A Civil War surgical "ace" might remove a leg in thirty seconds.

In 1846, the American dentist William Morton showed that diethyl ether could make a patient unconscious and allow a surgeon to operate at a more leisurely pace. Development and refinement of anesthesia techniques has gone on ever since. The ability to relieve pain allowed the surgeon more time to operate. Nevertheless, anesthesia as a separate medical discipline did not come into its own until after World War II. Before 1940, anesthesia could be administered by nearly any doctor or nurse. It was not a highly developed specialty.

> Anesthesia as a profession is a postwar phenomenon. Over the past fifty years the specialty of anesthesia has expanded to become one of the primary areas of modern medicine. Today, the profession's record of safety and effectiveness is remarkable.

To a modern-day anesthesiologist, prewar equipment seems primitive. The use of *muscle relaxants*, so common today, was also a wartime phenomenon. *Regional anesthesia* was in limited use. Today's sophisticated monitoring of the patient was unknown. There were even cases of injuries and deaths of both patients and doctors from explosions of flammable anesthetic agents. There were no recovery rooms.

By contrast, today's anesthesiologist works in an environment where every variable is under control. High technology abounds, and it's not just for show. Constant innovation—in drugs, monitoring, pain control, and recovery procedures — is the rule. Anesthesia deaths and mishaps cause quite a stir, but only because they are so rare. Going under anesthesia is far safer than driving to the hospital.

The field of anesthesia has had to expand and evolve. As surgery becomes more complex and pervasive, anesthesia has done an admirable job in keeping up. Today, despite the fact that medical (non-surgical) therapy is becoming increasingly prominent, the surgeon reigns supreme as the epitome of modern medicine; surgery patients occupy more than half of all hospital beds. None of this would have been possible without anesthesiology, which has become one of the most important specialties in medicine today. And it is important to note that, while the subject we treat here is surgical anesthesia, anesthesiologists have made great strides in a critical area unrelated to surgery, that of chronic pain control.

Anesthesia is not just one procedure or drug. Many kinds exist, each suitable for a different procedure. Anesthesia can often be tailored to fit both the surgery and the individual. Following are some of the terms you might hear.

## Local Anesthesia

*Local anesthetics* block pain transmission up the nerves that go to the spinal cord and the brain from the area being operated on. They can be used in different ways: *topically*, by *local infiltration, nerve block* and *regional*.

Local anesthetics are administered in several ways. One is by injection in the immediate area of surgery or somewhere along the major nerve serving the area. In hand surgery, for example, the anesthesia may be injected under the arm (an *axillary block*). For shoulder surgery, the injection will be higher up, in the neck (an *interscalene block*). These procedures together are known as *brachial plexus blocks*. Hand anesthesia can also be achieved by injecting local anesthetic into a hand vein while the circulation is halted by a tourniquet on the upper arm. This is called a *Bier block*.

Another method of administration uses a topical spray or drops for areas such as the eyes, throat, and the inside of the nose and mouth. In pediatrics, a skin ointment is now used for minor surgery and for preparing the child's skin for intravenous infusions.

The patient is fully conscious when local anesthesia is used alone. The surgical procedures for which local anesthesia alone is given are usually simple: removal of skin tumors, suturing of lacerations, dental work.

Sometimes local anesthesia may even be used at the patient's request in more complicated surgery. Some patients like to be alert and wide awake just to keep an eye on things. Dr. Jeanne Richardson of New York City used to hold up an automobile mirror to allow her conscious hernia patients to watch their own surgery. It's not every patient's cup of tea, but you may have the option.

Allergies to local anesthetics are rare. Most supposed allergies are really an overreaction to the *adrenalin* (*epinephrine*) that's sometimes used to constrict blood vessels in conjunction with the local anesthetic. It is possible, however, to react badly to an overdose of local anesthetics. These can cause convulsions or interfere with the heart function.

Local anesthetics are chosen according to their length of action. *Novocaine* and *lidocaine* are short-acting agents. Some longer-acting agents are *mepivacaine, bupivacaine,* and *tetracaine.*

## Local Supplemented with Sedation

*Sedation* is often used in conjunction with local anesthesia for several reasons. Sedation helps you feel more comfortable while you're being injected with the local anesthesia. Local anesthesia by itself does nothing to control nervousness (it can even increase it because of the use of epinephrine). Patients can be disturbed by the noise and activity of the operating room. Few people like the sound of their own bones being drilled. Sedation makes the patient feel calmer. Local infiltration of anesthesia is not profoundly numbing. And so the sedation helps blur sensations like touch, pulling, and pressure, making them easier for the patient to bear.

Commonly used sedatives are *diazepam, midazolam,* and *narcotics* like *meperidine, morphine,* and *fentanyl.* Low doses of intravenous anesthetics such as *sodium thiopentone* and *propofol* are also used.

## Regional Anesthesia

*Regional anesthesia* refers to anesthesia administered in the area of the spine. It was first tried in Germany in the nineteenth century, using cocaine. The purpose is to block transmission of pain impulses from the lower half of the body, through the spinal cord, to the brain. *Spinals* and *epidurals* are the two major types. As with local, regional anesthesia can be combined with sedation.

In a spinal, the injection of the anesthetic is made into the cerebral spinal fluid that surrounds the spinal cord in the lower part of the back. The anesthetic can't be injected any higher because the spine actually ends around the first lumbar vertebra.

Epidurals are given most commonly in the lower back. They can also be given in between the joints of the tailbone (the coccyx), and, more rarely, at locations on the upper spine and in the neck. What this amounts to is the carefully controlled injection of a local anesthetic into these areas. In the case of lumbar epidurals and spinals, the patient can be anesthetized from the abdomen down.

The chief advantage? You don't need general anesthesia. Surgeons who do knee and hip replacements feel that patients are less likely to develop clots in the legs that can travel up to the lungs. In obstetrics the mother can be conscious when the baby is born without feeling any pain. It's also safer for the baby. Many patients want to be conscious, either out of curiosity or out of fear of losing consciousness and control. There may be less postoperative pain because pain is blocked and never reaches the brain.

If you have an epidural, the anesthetic is injected through a needle in the epidural space. The epidural space is the area just outside the space surrounding the spinal cord (where a spinal would be given). Unlike the spinal space, the epidural space is not filled with fluid. Before removing the needle, the anesthesiologist often threads a little plastic tube (*epidural catheter*) through the needle into the epidural space. This can be used during surgery to add more anesthetic if needed. After surgery the tube can be used to administer narcotics. Narcotics administered this way result in profound pain relief with less sedation. But if you undergo this technique, you'll need special nursing care, so it is not always available.

Regional is also the technique of choice for some patients with multiple medical problems. If a patient has a serious heart or lung problem, the doctor may wish to avoid general anesthesia because of its effect on breathing or the heart. Surgeons often request spinal anesthesia for removal of the prostate gland (*transurethral resection of the prostate*) because there is less bleeding and better bladder relaxation.

New findings suggest that in certain instances patients may suffer from less postsurgical pain after regional than after general anesthesia. The reason: the patient's brain registers the pain under general anesthesia, even though the patient didn't seem to "feel" the pain at the time of surgery. Under regional, the pain impulse did not reach the brain in the first place, so the brain had no "pain memory."

## General Anesthesia

*General anesthesia* is a combination of intravenous medications and gases you breathe in that work together to act on the brain and cause unconsciousness. The patient is brought into an unconscious state in a controlled manner, with all vital functions carefully monitored.

General anesthesia slows or depresses breathing and heart function. As a result, measures need to be taken to assist or control the patient's breathing. Heart functions must also be monitored and may need to be supported with certain drugs and fluids.

*Muscle relaxants* are often used with general anesthesia. They make it easier to insert an *endotracheal tube* to protect the lungs from stomach contents and to control breathing. By relaxing certain muscles, they help surgeons work inside the abdomen. As a result, the patient can be carried on a relatively light (hence safer) level of anesthesia. Muscle relaxants do not affect consciousness or pain perception; they simply prevent movement.

No one really knows how general anesthesia works. From the surgeon's point of view, the patient seems to feel no pain. But the patient does react to the surgical invasion. The patient's pulse rate and blood pressure may increase. Signs of sweating, wrinkling of the brow, tension in the jaw muscles, tears—all may appear. These are signs for the anesthesiologist to increase the depth of anesthesia. At even lighter levels, if the patient's muscles aren't relaxed, the operating team would then see withdrawal movements.

After the surgery, the patient remembers nothing, but we know the brain is still responding to the painful stimulus of the surgery, even though the surgery is now over. If certain techniques are used to block the transmission of pain to the brain from the area being operated on, the patient uses less postoperative pain medication. This shows that there may be a long-term reaction to a painful stimulus even though it is not consciously perceived.

A good example involves amputated arms or legs. Patients may feel horrible *phantom* pain in their lost limbs for years. If the patient had pain on the limb before the amputation, they might still feel pain on the removed limb after surgery. The limb is no longer there to feel the pain; the pain comes from the brain instead. If, on the other hand, the painful stimulus never gets to the brain because of a *spinal* or *epidural* block, then phantom limb pain is much less likely. Naturally, the spinal or epidural cannot control the effect of pain felt before the surgery.

When is general anesthesia used? For operations such as open heart surgery; most pediatric surgery; head, neck, and throat surgery; operations on major body cavities such as lungs and abdomen; most brain surgery; organ transplants; and nearly any other type of surgery. Many patients will opt for general in circumstances where local is possible. They prefer to be "asleep" and unaware.

Drugs used intravenously are *sodium thiopentone*, *propofol*, muscle relaxants like *curare*, and narcotics like morphine and fentanyl. *Nitrous oxide* (laughing gas) is inhaled. Other inhalation agents such as *isoflurane*, *enflurane*, and *halothane* are vaporized and mixed with oxygen and nitrous oxide in a controlled manner. Newer agents are constantly being developed.

## A Bewildering Choice

In choosing your anesthetic, the surgeons, in conference with the anesthesiologist, have the final say. They, after all, know what conditions they require to perform the operation. But you, the patient, do have some input. It may not be possible to have local rather than general anesthesia, for example, but you owe it to yourself to ask about the options. Your anesthesiologist is there to help you make choices when you have them and to help you understand the procedures that will be used.

# Four

# Breakthroughs

*Art and science have their meeting point in method.*

Bulwer-Lytton

» Anesthesia became a true specialty only about fifty years ago. Since then, the pace of change has been rapid. New techniques are fast coming on line, while others are waiting in the wings. Some of these new techniques can spare us from pain, shorten our hospital stay, help us recover quickly, and even save us money. But this will happen only if they're used.

Some current or imminent breakthroughs:

• Narcotics can now be targeted directly to pain receptors to block pain, with fewer side effects. Narcotics placed in the knee and shoulder joints can bring pain relief for several days after arthroscopic surgery. Narcotics can also be placed around the spinal cord for similar results. As we shall see in later sections, pain can be "learned" and later reproduced. The new techniques prevent the potentially painful impulse from reaching the brain in the first place, so the brain can't "memorize" the pain and later reproduce it or even magnify it.

- Advances in pharmacology have given us new drugs like *ketorolac tromethamine*, a potent pain reliever that doesn't depress respiration.
- A whole new group of narcotics that don't depress respiration is being developed.
- *Desflurane* is a new anesthetic vapor that not only works more quickly, it leaves the body more quickly than other agents do, so that patients can go home earlier.

> Exciting breakthroughs in anesthesia and pain control are announced in nearly every medical journal that comes down the pike. Yet none of these new techniques can make up for a full, caring relationship between a concerned doctor and a well-informed patient.

- New research is investigating *artificial hibernation* agents which slow down metabolism to allow surgeons to operate on organs like the brain and heart.
- Research on the brain and emotions, combined with research on how pain is actually created and felt, has led to new psychological techniques to keep pain under control. Suggestion and relaxation tapes are coming into use more and more during surgery, as well as before and after. The net result is less pain, diminished fear, quicker healing, and a faster recovery.
- Doctors in Europe have found new uses for the familiar drug *hydergine*; it protects the brain from low oxygen levels during surgery.
- Computerized administration of medication is becoming more and more prevalent.

- Skin patches impregnated with the narcotic fentanyl are being used to provide pain relief without injections. Fentanyl in the form of a lollypop has even been used for small children.

- Monitoring devices keep making anesthesia safer and more effective. *Pulse oximetry*, which measures the oxygenation of the blood, and *capnography*, which measures the carbon dioxide coming out of the lungs, are now both standard in the operating room.

- New surgical techniques, which make smaller incisions, cause less pain and shorten the recovery time. An example is laparoscopic surgery. Here, fiber optic tubes travel into your body. They are attached to a video camera outside, which the surgeon uses to coordinate the operation. You can bring your own videotape so you can entertain your friends and neighbors later on with details of your surgery. It's probably more interesting than your last trip to Orlando.

These are only a small sampling of what's going on in anesthesia. Anesthesiologists, surgeons, pharmacologists, psychologists, hospitals, medical equipment manufacturers, and drug companies all have their effect on the pace of change and how new techniques are used in operating rooms. But these techniques are of no value if they aren't used.

# Five

# Who Will I Be Dealing With?

*Medicine is not only a science; it is also an art. It does not consist of compounding pills and plasters; it deals with the very processes of life, which must be understood before they may be guided.*

Paracelsus

» More than twenty-three million surgical procedures are performed in the United States annually. That averages to more than sixty-three thousand a day; or about forty-two every minute. Surgical personnel in America are among the world's finest, but, obviously, they are also among the world's busiest. We can and should assume that surgical personnel want to give you the best possible medical care. But your own input into the equation is crucial.

The key to success and a less painful postoperative experience is to take charge and assume nothing. This doesn't mean that you should become a nuisance to your surgeon, anesthesiologist, and nurses. It does mean that you should ask questions and request that modern pain control procedures be used, without fear of being seen as a nuisance. Remember, smart people ask "stupid" questions. In the heat of the moment, when a lot is going on, you can't count on remembering everything. Write your questions down and remain firm about having them answered.

## Who Makes the Pain Control Decisions?

The surgeon and anesthesiologist, preferably in conjunction with the patient, are the prime decision makers. Nurses, of course, are responsible for a significant amount of medication both before and after surgery. In some settings, a highly trained nurse-anesthetist may deal with pain control under the direction of a surgeon or anesthesiologist.

Your hospital may also have a pain management service that deals with both surgical and chronic pain. These are usually run by anesthesiologists.

All these professionals have a say in how you are medicated. They will decide which narcotics will be administered and in what dosages. Narcotic drugs can be addictive. They are often abused. But they do have a *proper place* in surgical and postsurgical pain control. Because fear of drug abuse and addiction in our society is so strong, you, the patient, cannot take for granted that you will receive the proper level of narcotics for pain relief. You must make it clear to all the personnel you deal with that you insist on truly effective pain control. You must make sure each understands what you have discussed with the others—no matter how rushed the setting.

Many new pain control drugs and procedures are coming into practice that do not use narcotics (and that do not depress respiration or make you groggy). *Ketorolac* and other *NSAIDs* (non-steroidal anti-inflammatory drugs) are examples. One disadvantage of NSAIDs is that they tend to increase bleeding. But narcotics are still the mainstay, with no true substitute. You still might have to swim upstream against a long-standing tendency of many professionals to under-medicate. Pervasive under-medication for postsurgical pain has resulted in a congressional inquiry.

## The Anesthesiologist

The preoperative phase of surgery (pre-op for short) can take many forms. In certain situations, you might be able to come into the hospital and meet with a member of the anesthesia department while you get your pre-op testing (lab tests, cardiograms, etc.). The anesthesiologist will review your history and find out about any special problems you might have had with anesthesia before. Here you'll let the anesthesiologist know if you're allergic to any type of anesthesia, if you're taking special medications, if you have diabetes, heart or lung problems, or other physical ailments that require special handling.

This is the time to get the question of anesthesia risk out of the way. Anesthesia is extremely safe; you take a greater risk by walking to the hospital. But because you are human, you will have concerns — about things major and minor. One thing you might worry about is getting a bad headache from a spinal anesthetic. The time to resolve such concerns is during your conference with the anesthesiologist — not the moment before surgery.

The preoperative interview is the time to decide what type of anesthesia you'll be receiving. You may be in a situation where there isn't much choice, or where you've already gone over the matter with the surgeon. But if you do have several choices, this is the time to talk about them.

One thing that concerns anesthesiologists is whether or not the patient smokes. Apart from the long-term damage, smoking before and after surgery will delay healing by impairing the immune system and by constricting the small blood vessels in the skin where healing takes place. This is especially important in cases of cosmetic surgery and skin grafts. Skin wound infections are more common in patients who smoke.

It may seem strange, but the anesthesiologist will want to assess the state of your teeth. Loose teeth that become dislodged may cause serious complications during anesthesia. If you have special dental work such as caps, the anesthesiologist should know in order to do his or her best to see that the dental work is not damaged.

> A full preoperative interview by your anesthesiologist is an essential part of the surgical experience. The doctor will explain medications and procedures and ask you important health questions. But you get your own turn while the doctor listens — to ask questions, to voice concerns, to make requests regarding your treatment and personal needs.

The anesthesiologist will also check out certain of your physical peculiarities such as a receding chin or a thick neck. Either can lead to difficulty in inserting a breathing tube.

The preoperative visit is a time for you to air your concerns with the anesthesiologist. If friends or members of your family have had previous unpleasant or dangerous experiences with anesthesia or anesthetics, this is the time to get it out in the open with the anesthesiologist. Clearing the decks of all the worries you have will help you in healing.

A leisurely pre-op interview may not be possible, however, even in the finest hospitals; there simply isn't enough time. Rather, the anesthesiologist may telephone you the night or morning before your operation to see how you're doing. In all cases the anesthesiologist will be fully familiar with the contents of your medical record. If there is no official preoperative anesthesia clinic at your hospital, you could call the anesthesia department to speak with an anesthesiologist. This would be especially helpful if you are coming into the hospital the same day of surgery.

The next step involves the period immediately before the operation. The anesthesiologist will prescribe an *intravenous infusion*. The intravenous is necessary for several reasons. The patient will have been fasting for awhile and needs extra essential fluids, especially in cases where there is going to be blood loss. Many of the anesthetic agents go directly into the circulation through the intravenous, avoiding the need for giving the patient constant injections.

Most patients will have been sedated also, before they go to the operating room. They'll have had a sedative either by mouth, such as *diazepam*, or more commonly an intramuscular or intravenous injection. Why sedation? The reasons are obvious: fear and anxiety can cause a dangerously rapid pulse and high blood pressure. These in turn make it harder for your body to respond to anesthesia. Sedation reduces the hazard. Many patients are also given medicine (antacids or anti-emetics) to prevent nausea and vomiting, which can be particularly dangerous during anesthesia.

It's standard procedure for various personnel to double- and triple-check *basic essentials* about the operation with the patient: which leg (or eye, or breast) is being operated on? Have you followed instructions not to eat anything? Do you have any allergies? These repetitive questions may drive you crazy, but they serve as necessary stopgaps to prevent surgical error.

The anesthesiologist will spend the fifteen minutes or so before you are wheeled into the operating room making a careful equipment check.

Although they may seem like cold and inhuman machines, you should think of these instruments of technology as your special friends and guardians. They'll give your doctor information about your body's reactions and condition. And they'll help the doctor make crucial decisions — often very quickly — about your care.

Let's get to know some of these buddies of ours:

- The *anesthesia gas machine* is the mainstay of the operating room. It's the primary source of anesthetics in gaseous form.

- The *ventilator* will pump oxygen and anesthesia gases to your lungs. In order to get them there smoothly, the anesthesiologist will often *intubate* you by placing an *endotracheal tube* into your windpipe after you are asleep.

- The *oxygen monitor* measures the amount of oxygen being delivered to you.

- A *standard electrocardiogram* monitor displays your heart rate and rhythm.

- A *sphygmomanometer*, the traditional blood pressure monitor, with its pressure cuff for the arm.

- A *body temperature monitor*. The probe will either be positioned in your esophagus or taped to your skin.

- A *pulse oximeter* calculates and displays the oxygen content in your blood through a sensor either placed on a finger or clipped to an earlobe.

- A *capnograph* measures exhaled carbon dioxide. It will warn the anesthesiologist if you are not breathing adequately and show immediately if the breathing tube is in the wrong place or has been accidentally disconnected.

- A *low pressure monitor* detects accidental disconnection of the anesthetic tubes running from the anesthesia machine to the patient.
- A *computerized pump* may be used to continuously administer minute intravenous dosages of anesthetics, according to the anesthesiologist's instructions. The anesthesiologist will program the machine before surgery to meet your particular needs. Of course, the settings can be changed by a manual override — like the cruise control in your car.
- A nerve stimulator to test the degree of muscle relaxation.
- Flexible pipes to the wall of the room to carry oxygen and nitrous oxide gas to the anesthesia gas machine from a hospital central supply. Backup tanks of the gases are attached to the machine, should the central supply fail.
- An anesthesia supply cart that contains all necessary drugs, plus the ones the anesthesiologist hopes will not be necessary but keeps ready for an emergency during the operation.

These are the basics. More and more operating rooms are linking all this equipment to a computer that can record each surgical event — the drug administered, the patient's reaction — for precise and total monitoring and record keeping.

In certain types of specialized surgery today, an *ultrasonic monitor* (or *echocardiogram*) may follow the movements of the heart, or a *Swan Ganz catheter* may be used to measure pressures inside the heart. A modified *electroencephalogram* (EEG) may be used to monitor brain activity. Although the EEG is still of limited use for monitoring depth of anesthesia, an experimental beginning has been made in this important area.

It now comes time for the actual administration of anesthesia. Before the you get to the operating room the anesthesiologist or a nurse inserts an intravenous line into the your arm. Once you are ready and the machinery has been checked out rigorously, the anesthesiologist takes your vital signs — pulse and blood pressure.

As soon as you come into the operating room, even as the first steps in the anesthesia are being accomplished, a monitoring process that will extend through the postoperative phase begins. All vital body functions are monitored: cardiogram, blood pressure (at least every five minutes), the level of oxygen in your blood, exhaled carbon dioxide, temperature. This is the time your anesthesiologist might ask you to think of some calming place you would rather be. This is the moment you go under.

Next, the anesthesiologist or nurse anesthetist administers a drug (such as propofol) to induce sleep and a narcotic (such as fentanyl) to act as a pain blocker. A muscle relaxant (such as *succinylcholine chloride*) may also be used for a short period in order to make it easier for the breathing tube to be inserted down the trachea.

The surgeon is still not at work. The anesthesiologist checks vital signs again, makes sure the patient is responding well to the anesthetics already administered, then begins to guide an endotracheal tube into the windpipe. This tube will serve as an important highway during the operation. Down it will travel varying combinations of oxygen, nitrous oxide, or vaporized anesthetics. The concentrations of these gases and vapors will be regulated to make the sleep-like state deeper or lighter, to make amnesia more complete, and to keep pain under control.

While the surgeon is at work, the anesthesiologist's main task is to monitor these functions, which can change in response to anesthesia and surgery, and to maintain the anesthetic state. (We'll be talking about awareness under anesthesia a little later, but for now assume that all this will go on without you knowing about it.)

The anesthesiologist's first task during the postoperative process is reversing the anesthesia. Reversal starts in the operating room and continues in the recovery room. In the recovery room you'll be handed over to the care of a nurse specially trained in taking care of patients recovering from surgery. The anesthesiologist is still available for monitoring the patient's stability: breathing, recovering alertness, comfort. Here also the anesthesiologist may confer with pain service personnel to make sure proper pain medications are maintained without interruption. In situations where no pain management service is available, the anesthesiologist may take on the role of postoperative pain manager. It should be noted that the anesthesiologist is highly qualified to do so, as most pain management services are run by anesthesiologists.

Remember that when you wake up in the recovery room there may be additional equipment attached to you that you didn't have before you went to sleep. If you do your homework on this there won't be any surprises. You could have a tube in your bladder or your nose, or the endotracheal tube might even still be in your throat. In addition to an intravenous you may have a tube in your artery or one going into your neck, for monitoring your arterial and venous blood pressure. There may also be drainage tubes coming from the area of the surgery. Dressing or casts round out the list. Something that many patients also find curious is the sticky feeling in their eyes. This is due to the protective eye ointment used during surgery.

## Nursing

Nurses play a very important role in providing care. Operating room nurses are very highly trained in advanced technology, but you may see them as being the kindest people that you meet. They keep the operating room running.

In many cases, the nurses become strong patient advocates. They will see that you are comfortable, that your belongings are taken care of, and that your needs are communicated to doctors. They are also concerned with maintaining hospital rules and regulations. It will be a nurse who checks that you are fully prepared for surgery: that you understand and sign your consent, that you have an empty stomach, that you are properly shaved.

> *There is so much emphasis on high tech in medicine today, that the personal touch can suffer. New and innovative approaches to communication between professionals and patients have to be developed. Nurses can form the critical link between the patient and the family while the patient is in the hospital. At my hospital, they are the ones who keep the family informed of the patient's progress during and after the surgery.*
>
> Michele Chotkowski, RN

Nurses also administer much of the medication you receive before and after the surgery. During local anesthesia, the nurse may sit with you, monitor your vital signs and keep you comfortable.

Most of your care in the hospital will be provided by nurses. They are important in relaying information between you and the doctors and they are always ready to help you.

# Six

# Smart People Ask Stupid Questions

*Wisdom is ofttimes nearer when we stoop than when we soar.*

Wordsworth

» Everyone has an area of expertise. If yours is anesthesia and pain control, then you really don't need this book. If it isn't, you'll have to be very careful not to be intimidated by the level of expertise and authority of the medical personnel you'll be dealing with. It can happen very easily without the doctor really intending it. You'll have to have the guts to ask a question even though it may sound "stupid," even though it may show your total ignorance of medical procedures. The anesthesiologist or surgeon may seem busy or distracted, but you must still insist on having your questions answered in enough depth to satisfy you.

A medical professional, like any skilled person, runs the risk of misjudging how much the patient actually knows or understands about the procedure to be done. The doctor depends on you for clues about what you need to know. A few technical terms here and there and first thing you know—your mind is blank. So stop and take a

deep breath. Take notes if you need to. Just remember —
the medical people were once in your shoes. They had to
have it all explained to them once.

Many patients know a great deal about medical procedures, especially if they've been operated on more than
once. They don't need as much orientation. But let's say
you do. Don't be concerned that you are boring a skilled
professional by asking that elementary facts be repeated.
The sympathetic doctor genuinely wants your questions,
at whatever level. The less sensitive doctor needs to be
forced to attend to your needs patiently, until you are
satisfied with the answers. In either case, being too shy to
ask is inappropriate.

Smart people ask stupid questions. It's best to ask them
nicely, calmly, with consideration for the doctor's busy
schedule, with the assumption that the doctor is more than
happy to reply in depth. If these ideal conditions don't
apply in your situation, you'll still have to ask, even if you
have to make a pest of yourself. In either case, you have
an absolute right to full knowledge of the medical procedures you will be going through. You also have an obliga-
tion to yourself to do whatever you must do to get the
information you need.

> There is simply no substitute for
> knowledge about your own surgi-
> cal and anesthetic experience.
> Without this knowledge, everything
> will be simply "done to you." With
> the knowledge, you'll truly be part
> of the experience. You can only
> gain by knowing.

So you're determined to ask the questions you must ask.
Well, what are they? Questions should be specific and to

the point. They should be clearly phrased so the anesthesiologist or surgeon can understand them and answer them effectively. And you must write them down beforehand. One prime example is, "How much pain can I be expected to have after surgery?" Types of surgery differ, and patients do too. Breast surgery, for example, is often not particularly painful. Many patients get by on one or two shots and a pain pill; others don't need any medication, but feel comforted knowing it's available. Everybody reacts differently.

In a stressful, busy situation, you might not remember every question you wanted to ask. Once written down, questions can then be rephrased and edited. It's not an empty exercise; its goal is to make the communication between you and the doctor as smooth as possible, so you can be properly informed. A good level of knowledge not only satisfies your desire to know, it also lifts your emotional state, and your level of confidence. It allows you to go into your surgery on the best possible footing.

But asking the questions is not the end product. You also need to remember and sort through the answers. Here it's wise to have a friend or relative with you who can help you keep everything straight. It is also useful to have someone objective with you to help weigh your options. Here, once again, it pays to have pencil and paper handy.

If you haven't yet gone out and sharpened a dozen pencils, let an example from real life guide you. Doctors at Montefiore Hospital in New York City made audiotapes of presurgical interviews between surgeons and patients. When the patients were later asked if they remembered discussing certain subjects in the interviews, most remembered only a fraction of the discussion. The patients were astonished when the tapes were played back. The lesson is that you have too much detail to remember. Write it all down!

# Seven

# Fear of Addiction

*The mere apprehension of a coming
evil has put many into a situation of
the utmost danger.*

Lucan

» Fear of addiction is a larger problem than addiction itself.
It impacts on one of the major issues this book raises — *the
question of unnecessary pain after surgery.*

Drug addiction is horrible in individuals. The social
problems it causes are unfortunate. Doctors, at least
during their training as interns and residents, see some of
the worst sides of the problem. For a young doctor to see
teenagers wheeled into an emergency room — stone-cold
dead from drugs — has to be a wrenching emotional experience. Since doctors have better access to narcotics
than many people, drug abuse is also a real problem in
their own profession. It is rare to find a doctor who does
not know, or know of, a colleague who has had a drug
problem. So it is understandable that when faced with the
choice of a narcotic for a patient, the doctor may be
tempted to "Just Say No," when the correct answer is
"Yes."

The question of pain control in hospital patients is a complicated one. The doctors need to control your pain and keep you as comfortable as possible. Against this, they balance the possibility of unwanted effects of the drugs: nausea, decrease in breathing rate, lowering of blood pressure and excessive sleepiness. When morphine is used for pain relief in an epidural or spinal it can sometimes cause itching and problems passing urine.

> Let's put fear of addiction in its proper place. If you don't have a problem with substance abuse now, you won't develop one in the hospital. The fear of addiction is the doctor's problem, not yours. Your problem is making sure that the doctor's fear doesn't cause you unnecessary pain.

**Fact:** The illicit use of narcotics—what we call drug abuse—has absolutely nothing to do with the proper use of these drugs: to relieve unbearable pain during and after surgery in the context of hospital care. The blanket prejudice against narcotics on the part of many doctors has resulted in much unnecessary pain. Remember, it is the patient who suffers the pain, not the doctor. Often, because of the authority and respect the doctor commands, the patient will suffer the pain in silence.

**Fact:** Drug addiction among surgical patients is extremely rare. The social and environmental factors that cause drug addiction on the streets are simply not present for the average patient in a hospital situation. Most people don't enjoy being stuporous. As we shall examine later on in this book, pain can be much more dangerous to the well-being of the patient than any drug, properly administered.

In experiments with PCA, or Patient-Controlled Analgesia, patients were allowed to press a button that tells a machine to give morphine to themselves whenever they thought they needed it (*analgesia* simply means a state of not feeling pain, although conscious). They consistently chose *less* medication than the doctor would have prescribed. The use of the narcotics for pleasure, for kicks, for escape, just didn't come up in the surgical setting. The practice of letting patients administer their own narcotics in this way is now widespread.

> *Don't worry about getting "hooked" on pain medicine. Studies show that this is very rare — unless you already have a problem with drug abuse.*
>
> U.S. Public Health Service, Agency for Health Care Policy and Research, ACPR Pub. No. 92-0021, Feb. 1992

Since addiction to narcotics in surgical patients is indeed rare, these drugs stack up well in terms of safety when compared with NSAIDs (nonsteroidal anti-inflammatory drugs) such as aspirin, acetaminophen, and ibuprofen. NSAIDs are available over the counter. When overused (and they are) they can cause nausea, stomach bleeding and kidney problems. Worse, they are simply not strong enough to take care of heavy-duty surgical pain. So there are lots of advantages to using narcotics.

In no case, however, is surgery totally free from discomfort. If you expect narcotics to completely eradicate all pain, you may be disappointed. But you can expect them to keep pain to a manageable level.

The well-informed patient has several tasks regarding narcotic drugs. The first is to ascertain the doctor's attitudes. Begin by simply asking the doctor about his or her feelings on using narcotics. If the doctor seems to have an unreasonable or inflexible prejudice against narcotics, it may be wise to bring in someone from the pain control service to add a second opinion. The second task, now that you have learned more about pain control, is to demand that the doctor give you appropriate levels of medication and then carefully monitor your pain. Toughing it out is not the right strategy for modern medicine. The modern pain control specialist has the knowledge to ensure that the level of medication given is neither too little nor dangerously high. Today's properly informed patient has the responsibility to insist on getting the right level of medication.

# Eight

# The Surgeon

> *Excellence, in any department, can only be attained by the labor of a lifetime. It is not purchased at a lesser price.*
>
> Samuel Johnson

» Today's surgeons are wonderfully skilled and usually highly specialized. Of course the surgeon knows a thing or two about anesthesia and pain control, but it's not the main focus. The surgeon does care if you undergo pain, but you pay the surgeon for technical ability and medical judgment. The surgeon has experience in diagnosing your problem, in choosing the correct treatment, in knowing when to operate, and in knowing how to operate. The surgeon's bedside manner is secondary.

The surgeon will serve as your first lead to the personnel who will be responsible for your anesthesia and pain management. The anesthesiologist is the pain control specialist and may have to act as your pain control advocate with the surgeon. Additional pain service personnel may also be there to help you.

Here's a critical fact to keep in mind. During the actual surgery, the anesthesiologist is the one who keeps watch over the patient. The anesthesiologist not only watches the anesthetic state, but supports your breathing and other vital functions. The surgeon is there to concentrate on the surgery.

Of course, surgeons differ as to their approach. A surgeon conversant with modern techniques, like micro incisions, can leave you with a lot less wear and tear on your body. The right surgeon can make your surgical experience less of a burden, your hospital stay shorter, and the job of the anesthesiologist easier. While many exciting techniques are still experimental, some have become routine. Nearly eighty percent of the six hundred thousand gallbladder operations done each year, for example, are performed with laparoscopes and video monitoring. Four tiny punctures through the skin act as ports for the surgical instruments used in operating on the gallbladder. Formerly, a much larger incision had to be made in the abdomen. With the modern technique, the patient stays in the hospital overnight, rather than a week. But micro surgery is not always possible, and the surgeon is always ready to make a larger, conventional incision if the case demands it.

> Surgeons today are simply superb, but let them concentrate on their specialties. Pain control is up to the anesthesiologist and supporting staff; even more, it's up to you.

It's up to you to ask your surgeon about the kind of techniques that can make your surgery more successful and less painful. Don't assume that the surgeon expects one of your main concerns to be postsurgical pain. The surgeon's job is diagnosing the problem, planning the surgery, and getting you well. These are important areas for you to learn something about. But you can and should also bring up pain management. You can tell the surgeon you want to consider PCA or epidural narcotics, if appropriate. It's all part of becoming fully informed about all your options.

Today, the surgeon is quite an authority figure. The surgeon's words carry a lot of weight. It's important for you to keep in mind that the surgeon is an authority on surgery. The surgeon can give you statistics about healing. But the surgeon is not an authority on the individual's (your) ability to heal yourself. In Dr. Furlong's anesthesia practice, she discourages surgeons from telling patients, "It's going to hurt like hell." They may mean well, but they may also implant negative thoughts in the patient's mind. The surgeon's words can cut as deeply as their scalpels. Dr. Furlong tries to get surgeons on the side of promoting the patient's success, rather than being pessimistic.

# Nine

# Pain as a Learned Phenomenon

*As an enemy is made more fierce when we flee, so Pain grows proud to see us knuckle under it. She will surrender upon much better terms to those who stand and fight against her.*
Montaigne

» Canadian psychologist Ronald Melzack is one of the great pioneers in pain research. A truly innovative scientist, Melzack began experiments with newly weaned Scottish terriers. He deprived them of sensory stimuli for a time, then let them loose to see how they reacted. Strangely, *until they learned better*, the puppies showed none of the ordinary signs of pain that they should have; naturally curious, they would even stick their noses into a flame to see what was going on.

Melzack's subsequent work led to a radical change in how scientists view pain, and a greater respect for pain as a complicated phenomenon. Pain is neither physical or psychological; it can't be so easily pigeonholed. The brain, according to Melzack, doesn't just register the pain, it "creates" the pain. Even more startling, but accepted today, is the notion that the brain "creates" the body. Patients who have broken their spinal-cords completely often still can feel their body below the point of the break. The reason: the body areas they feel are still represented in the brain. How else could a person feel acute chronic pain in a limb that had been amputated years before? According to Melzack, the path from the source of the injury to the brain is not straight, as had been believed, but has *gates* that act to control the pain signals.

Following Melzack's gate theory, pain signals pass through the open gates in the spinal cord on their way up to the brain. Sharp pains are quicker. They register first, through one set of nerve fibers. They are followed by slower, duller aches that travel through other sets of fibers.

The communication, however, is two way. The brain sends messages back down to the gates. The gates will then either open up or close down, depending on the message. If this theory is indeed true, it shows how pain is indeed a perception of the brain. The brain is not forced to accept the pain impulse in every instance. It can close the gates. It often does.

In the real world, outside the laboratory, the pragmatic result of this breakthrough is straightforward: *pain felt is pain learned.* It's a ripple effect. Once the cycle of pain is begun, the pain will have a tendency to remain and increase. We are used to ordinary pain in our everyday lives, but in surgery, pain which we are not used to can be devastating. The shock is to our system — mind and body — as a whole. Physical, mental, emotional, and psychological feelings all mix together to create disequilibrium, a potentially dangerous state. Phantom pain, especially the long-term variety, is one of the worst manifestations of learned pain. But there are others, and if we want to control pain, we have to be on guard against the part of our thinking process which cooperates with or even creates pain.

In a heightened, over-sensitized state, we become overly vulnerable to new pain; we react to it badly. Surgical healing is impaired. Our general health suffers. Pain can depress the immune system and make you more likely to get an infection. Pain can make it harder to breathe, increasing the risk of pneumonia or a heart attack. Pain can make you sleep badly. Pain can make you exhausted and depressed. Pain can be a pain.

That's why it's critically important not to let pain in the front door, not to "learn" pain. During surgery, the use of music and suggestion tapes has proven effective in many cases in guiding the patient through the experience without "learning" the pain. Presurgery relaxation exercises, both mental and physical, are also helpful. Even though the patient may be under general anesthesia, modern research, as we shall later see, recognizes that sensation and hearing may still occur. Once the violent invasion of the body is sensed by the brain, even if the patient is too heavily drugged at the time to exhibit the usual reactions to pain, potential harm can occur.

Melzack's view of pain is that it's multidimensional. Pain isn't just a measurable series of electrical or chemical impulses. It also has emotional and cognitive dimensions. Since the brain is the key to it all, messages that come *from the brain* can balance or negate the pain messages that head from the source of the pain *to the brain*. This explains why in situations of great excitement or mental activity (a soldier in combat or an athlete in the middle of an event for example), a person can sustain a wound or injury without knowing it — the pain has been temporarily blocked. Once the activity ends, some minutes after the injury, the pain may be felt or learned for the first time. At that point the pain might snowball from insignificant to excruciating.

Pain lets us know the body has been injured so we can then do something to prevent further injury. That's the purpose of pain. Pain began as a survival instinct. But Melzack also found that much pain has little survival value. The pain may be way out of proportion to the tissue damage it's meant to warn us of. Instead, the pain has become a habit, a bad habit.

> The Gate Theory of pain looks at pain as a complex series of neurological events. Since the brain "creates" the body's pain — the brain can also protect the body from pain.

Chronic pain is not the subject of this book, but there is a lesson to be learned from Melzack's research on it. Pain is a powerful and mysterious force that can take on a life of its own. During surgery, we need to use every weapon we have to keep pain from taking us over. The body, it seems, has its own natural opiate receptors and opiates. Drugs such as morphine fit into the receptors the way a key fits into a lock, creating a defensive wall against pain. Unnecessary surgical pain, however, punches great holes in our pain defenses. It weakens us in mind, body, and spirit. For this reason, unnecessary surgical pain is more than just a temporary inconvenience, it's a fundamental menace to our health and well-being.

Anesthesiologists are using drugs that work directly on the spinal cord to close pain gates at critical times during the surgery. It has become clear to many physicians who treat pain that the timing of medication is just as important as the dose. A medication that blocks the worst pain at just the right moment will keep the patient's brain from dwelling on — learning — the pain.

Melzack himself has been a great campaigner for wider use of opiates, citing particularly the devastating pain suffered by children and cancer patients. He stresses that when people with psychological problems are screened out, opiate addiction or abuse is extremely rare. Even patients who are given the ability to choose their dosages rarely do so unnecessarily, despite the fact that opiates can be pleasurable. Normal surgical patients are oriented toward relief, not "kicks."

The message to you as a patient is clear. Respect pain and what it can do to you. But also respect your own ability to take active steps to keep the pain from reaching your control center —your wonderful brain—in the first place. You can, and should, make every effort to take charge of controlling your pain. In the next section, we'll outline a proven method of doing it.

# Ten

# Taking Charge

*Worry — a god, invisible but omnipotent. It steals the bloom from the cheek and lightness from the pulse; it takes away the appetite, and turns the hair gray.*

Benjamin Disraeli

» You can take charge of much of your surgical experience. The goal: leave as little as possible to chance. You can't control everything, but there's a lot you can do. We'll first speak about the hospital experience in general, then get specific about pain control issues.

## General Issues: Procedure/Surgeon/Hospital

If you're hit by a truck and are rushed to the hospital for emergency surgery, you don't have much time for trepidation. You may not even be awake. But most surgery is elective; you have choices to make and time to think. The waiting can be emotionally trying. You know you should study and plan, yet you become a jellyfish.

Knowledge — and plenty of it — is the cure for fears founded on ignorance. You may want to get a second opinion, but you have to be careful. The first opinion could very well be correct, the second wrong. The second opinion may also cost you money. Many insurers have determined that paying for second opinions doesn't really save them money (by avoiding unnecessary surgery), so they may not give coverage. So whether or not you go for a second opinion is a judgment call. It's up to you.

In a sense, any time you go to a surgeon it's always for the second opinion. *Your* opinion after your doctor says you need surgery is actually the first opinion. Your gut reaction, combined with a well-thought-out analysis of the realities and options of your situation, should guide you.

As an example, one of Dr. Furlong's patients was given a couple of options for her pervasive stomach problems. She could modify her diet and lifestyle or she could have surgery. After some thought, she decided that surgery was far easier than giving up the food she loved.

> Banking your own blood for your safe use during surgery is becoming more of an issue in these days of AIDS. You'll also have to determine how much blood you'll need. You'll need to research the issue and resolve it to your satisfaction.

If the surgery could be life threatening, you must face this possibility. The issue of living wills is controversial, but living wills do make sense. You may want to decide when and under what circumstances you should be kept alive artificially. This is the kind of thing that should be written down. Knowledge can only help you here; avoiding the issue may cause pain and suffering to both you and your family. Your surgery will probably go without a hitch, but the knowledge that you have provided for emergencies can still help you get through with a lower level of anxiety.

You must also sign a consent form before surgery. It's best to do this a few days ahead of time. No one wants to be told the worst possible scenario right before anesthesia.

## Pain Control — What You Can Do

The Federal Agency for Health Care Policy and Research sets out a seven step program to allow you to exercise maximum control over your own surgical pain. We have used these guidelines as the basis for the detailed program below.

BEFORE SURGERY

**STEP ONE:** ASK THE DOCTOR OR NURSE WHAT TO EXPECT.

• Will there be much pain after surgery?

• What will it feel like?

• Where and when will it occur?

• Why?

• How long is it likely to last?

Being prepared helps put you in control. You may want to write down your questions before you meet with your doctor or nurse.

**STEP TWO:** Discuss the pain control options that are available to you before, during, and after surgery.

Options before surgery will involve both drug and non-drug treatments. Common non-drug treatments involve relaxation exercises and deep breathing, but also ice or heat and massage.

During surgery, of course, you must receive some kind of anesthetic, but you can supplement the drug treatment with music, suggestion tapes or other non-drug adjuncts.

After surgery, both drug and non-drug options are available. The non-drug route might involve massage, hot or cold packs, relaxation, music or other pastimes to distract you, positive thinking, or nerve stimulation. We'll be discussing some of these techniques later on.

**Be sure to:**

● Talk with your nurses and doctors about pain control methods that have worked well or not so well for you before.

● Talk with your nurses and doctors about any concerns you may have about pain medicine.

● Tell your doctors and nurses about any allergies you may have to medicines.

● Ask about side effects that may occur due to the treatment.

● Talk with your doctors and nurses about the medicines you take for other health problems. The doctors and nurses need to know, because mixing some drugs with some pain medicines can cause problems.

> The average doctor at an office visit listens to the patient for eighteen seconds before interrupting. It's the well-informed patient's task to insist that this period be stretched out to at least a minute. Otherwise you're simply not making your needs known.

**STEP THREE:** Talk about the schedule for pain medicines in the hospital.

Some people get pain medicines in the hospital only when they call the nurse to ask for them. Sometimes there are delays, and the pain gets worse while they wait.

Today, two other ways to schedule pain medicines seem to give better results.

• Giving the pain pills or shots at set times. Instead of waiting until pain breaks through, you receive medicine at set times during the day to keep the pain under control. This tends to keep drug levels built up, ready to strike down pain, should pain arise. Some drugs take time to build up in the body to a level at which they're really effective.

• Patient-controlled analgesia (PCA) may be available in your hospital. With PCA, you can give the pain medicine to yourself. You don't have to ask a nurse or doctor for help. When you begin to feel pain, you press a button to inject the medicine through the intravenous (IV) tube in your vein.

For both ways, your nurses and doctors will ask you how the pain medicine is working. They'll change the medicine, its dose, or its timing, if you are still having pain.

**STEP FOUR:** Work with your doctors and nurses to make a pain control plan. The plan should be written down. It should cover presurgery, postsurgery, and at-home plans of what you will be taking and when. The medical personnel need your help to design the best plan for you. Once the plan is on paper, you'll be able to refer to it after your operation. Then keep it as a record if you need surgery in the future.

AFTER SURGERY

**STEP FIVE:** Take (or ask for) pain relief drugs when pain first begins.

● Take action as soon as the pain starts.

● If you know your pain will worsen when you start walking, doing breathing exercises, or physical therapy, take pain medicine first. It's harder to ease pain once it had taken hold.

**This is a key step in proper pain control.**

**STEP SIX:** Help the doctors and nurses "measure" your pain.

● They may ask you to rate your pain on a scale of zero to ten. Or you may choose a word from a list that best describes the pain.

● You may also set a pain control goal (such as having no pain that's worse than a two on the scale).

● Reporting your pain as a number helps the doctors and nurses know how well your treatment is working and whether to make any changes.

> Some people are predisposed to handling pain better than others. If you have a problem with pain, get to know your pain, learn to describe it accurately, and don't be shy about asking for relief.

**STEP SEVEN:** Tell the doctor or nurse about any pain that won't go away.

● Don't worry about being a "bother."

● Pain can be a sign of problems with your operation.

● The nurses and doctors want and need to know about the pain you experience.

You need to tell the nurses and doctors about your pain and how the pain control plan is working. They can change the plan if your pain is not under control.

Eleven
=

# Pain Management Credentials

*For fate has wove the thread of life with pain.*

Homer

➤ Even ten years ago, true pain management services could only be found in a few innovative hospitals in big cities. In the past few years, more and more doctors have come to realize how damaging pain can be to the well being of their patients. Pain management services are proliferating. More important, perhaps, is the fact that physicians now know about these services and make use of them.

So the pain management expertise is out there, no matter where you live. If you're looking at surgery, make sure every professional who treats you is well aware of the pain issues involved. Every modern hospital where surgery is performed should have a pain management service. If your hospital does not provide such a basic service as a distinct department, the anesthesia department will be your best resource for information about pain management.

Starting with *first* things, here's a useful checklist:

- Is your surgeon at least familiar with modern pain control techniques? Does the surgeon show a willingness to become familiar with your options for managing your pain?

- Does the hospital have a separate pain management service? If so, does it deal with surgical pain, chronic pain, or both? Is the pain management service accessible to you so you can ask it direct questions and not have to go through your doctor?

- Is the hospital's anesthesia department known for using state-of-the-art pain control techniques?

> We keep returning to the word "ask." If you persevere in asking the right questions, sooner or later you will get the information you need. But that's not enough. You must also ask that the treatment you need—modern, state-of-the-art pain treatment and nothing less—be given to you. You must ask, then ask again. As always, you must assume nothing.

- Does either the surgeon or the anesthesiologist seem to have a prejudice against using narcotics? Does there seem to be a reluctance to use narcotics in the hospital in general?

- Does the nursing staff seem to be on the ball regarding pain control? Do they work closely with the pain management service?

- Do the local agencies that monitor your hospital have a higher than normal level of complaints about surgical pain issues?

  *In any setting, the quality of pain control will be influenced by the availability of a pain management program and the training, expertise, and experience of its members. There is a wide variation among institutions in size, complexity, volume of surgical procedures, and differing patient populations; therefore, different pain management programs are suitable.*

  U.S. Public Health Service, Agency for Health Care Policy and Research, ACPR Pub. No. 92-0032, Feb. 1992

Your surgeon and anesthesiologist — in fact every doctor and nurse you deal with — should be able to satisfy your curiosity about the above and other questions you might have. If they don't seem fully conversant with modern pain control procedures — or worse, if they don't have time to answer your questions in the first place because they don't seem important — you can and should look elsewhere.

# Twelve

# Medicine and its Alternates

*Faith and knowledge lean largely upon each other in the practice of medicine.*

Peter Mere Latham

» We hear a great deal about *alternative* medicine. In some ways the term *alternative* is not accurate, because it implies that the patient has to choose between a conventional and an alternate treatment. Some people prefer to use the term "complementary medicine." The choice is not always either/or. As we use it here, the term *alternative* refers to healing techniques not generally associated with doctors and hospitals, though many doctors are coming to use them.

To most of us in the Western world, many of the alternative concepts are foreign. Some techniques may be used to treat a disease or symptom. Others are designed to enhance general health and resistance to disease. Many techniques focus on relieving stress and are useful when preparing for surgery.

Physicians have often been skeptical of alternative techniques. They feel they may cause patients to put off seeking help to deal with life-threatening problems such as cancer or coronary artery disease. They are justified to an extent. But doctors are also coming to realize that their conventional techniques have certain limitations. More and more they are using alternative techniques as an important supplement.

The issue of protecting the public is complex. In the future we will probably see many therapies we now call *alternative* becoming mainstream, even to the extent of being approved by government agencies. Under the leadership of Dr. Joseph Jacobs, the National Institutes of Health in Washington, D.C. opened an Office of Alternative Medicine in October 1992 to study and regulate these techniques. Insurance companies are also becoming more receptive to covering alternative therapies.

To better understand alternative medicine, it's useful to define what we mean by conventional medicine. Conventional medicine tends to rely on laboratory tests that express results in numerical form. Complicated and expensive equipment can be involved: radioactive tracers, CAT scans, ultrasound, to name a few. The patient has little involvement in finding and treating the problem, other than passively taking the doctor's advice. Many of the treatments have negative effects. Drugs may bring unwanted side effects.

Surgery, radiation, and chemotherapy are uncomfortable and stressful. Conventional medicine is also illness-oriented and does little to enhance the immune system and prevent disease. With the exception of a few major diseases like diabetes and heart disease, there is little emphasis on diet and lifestyle. For mental illness, the emphasis is on drug therapy.

By contrast most alternative techniques call for active patient participation. Treatments bring subtle changes and don't always work immediately. On the other hand, side effects are less prevalent. Many treatments work to build up the immune system or bring on a general feeling of well-being. Many increase the patient's feeling of autonomy. One important difference is that practitioners spend about twice as much time with their patients on the first visit as conventional doctors do.

While not often covered by insurance, alternative techniques are usually much less expensive; one reason is that they don't call for astonishingly expensive pieces of equipment like MRI (Magnetic Resonance Imaging) scanners. Practitioners are more likely than mainstream doctors to recommend dietary and lifestyle changes.

Access to alternative techniques varies with your location. Certain practitioners may not be licensed to practice in your area. But many alternative techniques come under the category of self-help, freely available everywhere. You can use many of the techniques below yourself. Some of the techniques have origins in ancient times.

Of course, there are points of crossover between mainstream Western medicine and alternative techniques. Relaxation for stress management, for example, is prescribed side by side with pills to control blood pressure and heart problems. A patient trained in techniques such as Lamaze and self-hypnosis for childbirth may elect to have an epidural injection of anesthesia as an adjunct to this training when the time comes to deliver.

## Acupuncture

In modern medicine our knowledge of the body is based on anatomical and microscopic dissection. The physiology is based on what we can see: the digestive system, the circulatory system, and so on. Traditional Chinese medicine explains the human body in an entirely different way, but with treatments that seem to work just as well. For example, the Chinese have the concept of *chi*. *Chi* is an energy force flowing throughout the body along certain meridians. It has qualities called *yin* and *yang*, which always oppose each other. The foods we eat and the herbs the Chinese use as medicines have corresponding yin and yang qualities. A traditional Chinese doctor will use acupuncture, change of diet, herbs, and exercises such as *tai chi* to manipulate the *chi* and achieve a balance or harmony. As odd as this system may seem to the Western mind, it works for millions of Chinese.

As one Chinese doctor now practicing in New York remarks, "In China I practiced mostly Western medicine, but now that I live in America I practice only Chinese medicine." The doctor has used acupuncture to control pain while orthopedic surgeons work on pinning bone fractures. This cuts down on the level of anesthesia needed and promotes bone healing. The patient has less pain and goes home earlier. Anesthesiologist André Clavel in New York has used acupuncture on the wrist to treat postoperative nausea. One group of anesthesiologists at Columbia University demonstrated the effectiveness of acupressure, using beaded wrist bands to prevent postoperative nausea and vomiting in cesarian section patients. While it was more popular in the nineteen seventies, acupuncture is now rarely used in hospitals. As interest in holistic treatments increases, however, acupuncture will probably come into wider use as an adjunct to anesthesia and pain management.

## Massage

The beneficial effects of massage have been known since ancient times. Massage has its place next to modern medical treatment as well. Recent research by Dr. Tiffany Field of the Miami Touch Research Institute has shown that the process of massage can help the person giving the massage as well as the person getting the massage. The immune function improves in both parties.

Whenever Dr. Furlong visits a friend in the hospital she always takes a little bottle of oil for back and hand or foot massages. More and more nurses are giving massages or encouraging visitors to do the same. Some nursing schools have had courses in healing touch for many years. With medicine so "high-tech," it's encouraging to run into examples of such "high-touch" activities.

## Nurses and Nurturing

Along with massage and other high-touch activities, more and more nurses are being encouraged to express their nurturing qualities. The Planetree concept, created by a hospital patient, has spurred a growing movement to change hospital environments. Planetree Units in San Francisco, in New York's Beth Israel Medical Center, and in Columbia, Oregon, retain the high-quality standards of conventional medicine, but with a more open environment. The nurse is likely to sit with the patient and give a comforting massage. Charts are accessible to the patients; the patient may even write in the chart. There is a kitchen where patients and relatives can prepare food just like back home. Close relatives of the patients are also encouraged to ask as many questions as they wish and to stay and visit as often as they like, even overnight. There is singing, music, poetry, and art. Central to the Planetree concept is the idea that the whole family should be involved in a person's illness and a recovery.

## Herbal Remedies

Dr. Furlong has never seen any herb prescribed in a hospital. They are not considered medicines, despite the fact that many of our modern medicines come from natural sources. Aspirin, for example, originally came from the willow bark. Morphine is made from opium, which comes from poppies. Digitalis comes from the foxglove plant. A major muscle relaxant used by anesthesiologists, curare, had its start as a poison used by South American Indians to tip their arrows. Part of the concern for the rain forests of South America is the possible permanent loss of valuable plant species with medicinal properties. Even mushrooms, such as the shiitake, have been shown to have immune-enhancing properties.

Why do we not use more of these remedies in hospitals? Partly because hospitals don't keep herbologists on staff. Producers of herbal medicines can't afford the 100 million dollars or so it takes to get a new drug approved by the federal Food and Drug Administration. Undoubtedly the FDA serves an important role in protecting the public from potentially harmful drugs, like thalidomide. But given the obvious value of many herbal substances, a new regulatory approach is needed to bring valuable herbs into wider medical use. The more effective the weapons we have in combating pain and enhancing healing, the better.

## Homeopathic Medicine

Homeopathy is a system of medicine begun by Samuel Hahnemann (1755-1843). Hahnemann believed that the symptoms of a disease are merely evidence of curative processes within the human body. Homeopathic doctors use certain substances (often minerals, herbs and plants) to accelerate the body's process of curing itself. Hahnemann found that certain substances taken in large amounts produced physical symptoms which mimicked different kinds of diseases. If he matched the symptom produced by the substance with a specific disease, then gave the patient the substance in a highly diluted form, the body would be stimulated to heal itself. Homeopathy was quite popular during the nineteenth century and is undergoing a revival today. In Britain, for example, forty percent of all physicians report referring patients to homeopathic practitioners; treatments are covered by the British National Health Service.

It's clear that homeopathy can be an excellent adjunct to conventional techniques. The aim: to enhance immunity and promote healing. Conventional doctors who use homeopathic techniques do so because they seem to work, even though they don't always know why. Some surgeons, for example, are using the alpine herb Arnica — available over the counter at health stores — to promote healing of wounds and fractures.

Dr. Jason W. Kwee, a Texas anesthesiologist who also practices homeopathy and acupuncture, explains that conventional doctors don't believe in homeopathy primarily because the substances used are so dilute. But homeopathic practitioners believe the dilution level makes the medicine even more powerful. Dr. Kwee uses the alpine herb *Arnica* in what he calls the "30 c" potency. He puts five or six drops under the tongue just before the patient wakes up. He has used this for hysterectomy and cesarian section patients. Dr. Kwee has found that many of these patients have a reduced need for narcotics, allowing some to take only acetaminophen. The surgeons he works with notice that, in many cases, wound healing seems to go faster. Dr. Kwee sometimes recommends that patients use Arnica for two days both before and after surgery for wound healing and pain reduction.

One of the major benefits of homeopathic substances is that they have no known toxicity. Used intelligently, they can provide valuable backup to conventional pain control and healing techniques.

## Meditation

Meditation is one of the most powerful stress relievers known. It typically consists of resting quietly and using some kind of technique to quiet the mind. The meditative state can also be induced by activities such as running, cycling, and walking: the repetitive rhythmical activity induces a calm and rested mind. Similar mental states can also be induced by chanting or by listening to music like Gregorian or Tibetan chants. The brain waves slow down and become more synchronized. *Endorphins*, the body's own natural sedatives, are released. Meditation also appears to change the way the body reacts to the stress hormones *adrenaline* and *noradrenaline*.

A simple meditation technique anybody can do is to rest quietly for twenty minutes and repeat a word over and over. The word could be meaningless or you could use a word that has deep meaning for you, as long as it concentrates and relaxes the mind. *Relax* and *Peace* are two good choices. Do this twice daily. The result will be an increased feeling of well-being, calmness, and a slowing of the pulse and breathing rate. Many people also meditate by finding a quiet place and staring at a flickering candle flame or mandala. Books, cassette tapes, and organized groups to help you meditate are fairly easy to find.

Everyone can benefit from meditation, in every aspect of life, but it's especially useful as a relaxation element before surgery. To use meditation to help get yourself through surgery does take some planning and practice beforehand, but the results are worth it. Once you feel the benefits of meditation, you'll probably continue with it long after you leave the hospital. It not only eases surgical pain, but it's very effective in working on chronic pain as well.

## Hypnosis and Visualization

There is a lot of misinformation out there about hypnosis. It's neither sleep nor a state of being under the power of another person. It's more a *natural* state of mind in which the lines of communication between the conscious and subconscious parts of your mind have been made exceptionally clear. Because of this, you are more susceptible than usual to the suggestions your subconscious mind receives—either from yourself or from a trusted therapist. Because the state of hypnosis is one of *enhanced* consciousness, you can't be induced to do anything you don't want to. Because the mind becomes clear, you may be able to bring back memories that previously were "buried." Hypnosis can also be used to erase a memory or resolve the conflicts in a memory.

Dr. Herbert Spiegel of Columbia University devised a simple technique that anybody can learn for inducing a state of hypnosis. He observed that some people are more receptive to being hypnotized than others. In order to have surgery without anesthesia you would need to be able to go into a deep trance. To completely relieve severe pain without drugs after surgery you would need to go into a trance slightly less deep. Not everybody can get that deep. But all of us can use hypnosis (or self-hypnosis) to relax and imprint useful healing concepts in the mind before or after surgery. Only a light to average level of hypnosis is necessary.

Here's a technique you can try during the days and weeks before your operation. Roll your eyes upward into your head as far as you can. Take a deep breath. As you breathe out, slowly close your eyes and tell yourself to relax. Tell yourself you are becoming more and more relaxed. You are learning to relax at will. You are also relaxing the muscles around the area of your operation. The more you learn to relax these muscles, the less discomfort you will have. You may also imagine a warm healing feeling in the area.

While in this relaxed state you can think of one hand being in a bucket of ice cold water. When the hand feels cold, place it on the part that hurts and transfer the diminished sensation there. This helps reduce swelling. Or you can just imagine a cool feeling in the sore place.

In some types of operations, such as skin grafts and muscle flaps, the doctor will need more blood to travel to the area. So imagine warm sunlight shining on the area. It's possible to redirect the flow of blood to different parts of the body through imagination. Tell yourself to move blood *away* from the surgical site during surgery, then *back* when the bleeding has been controlled and blood is needed for healing.

Now is also a good time to imagine being in the recovery room, feeling comfortable and relieved. The hospital stay seems short and going home is a happy time. Imagine simple things such as a nice family meal or vacation.

Hypnosis is a natural state. You don't need a bearded psychoanalyst with an Austrian accent dangling a watch in front of you. Even daydreaming can act as hypnosis if you daydream about the right things.

## Relaxation

Relaxation means different things to different people. It can be active or passive. You can relax by listening to music, watching TV, dancing, snuggling with a loved one, or walking on the beach. Or perhaps you relax by cooking, playing the piano, spending time with a pet. Anything you do that makes you feel good can help in the release of endorphins, the body's natural relaxants.

Some people find relaxation tapes useful to guide them to a relaxed state. Many of these tapes are available. Most of them guide you through a process of relaxing your body, one part at a time. Not everyone responds to these techniques. If you don't, or if these tapes make you irritable, don't worry; you have plenty of other ways to relax. Some people are also concerned about falling asleep while they are listening to a relaxation tape. But you shouldn't worry about that; falling asleep probably means the relaxation is working well.

Patients who concentrate on relaxing the muscles in the area of their surgery are able to reduce their postoperative pain and the amount of medicine they need. It helps to reach a generally relaxed state throughout your body first. But how do we relax the specific muscles? It's not hard. For example, if you're having breast surgery, you could start by identifying the muscles under the breast by tensing your arm against a chair, then releasing the tension. Soon the muscle is able to relax at will. It's a matter of getting in touch with your body.

Say you have abdominal surgery. After the operation, while lying in bed, use both your arms instead of your abdominal muscles to carry the weight of your body. This, as well as deeply relaxing the abdominal muscles, will greatly reduce the amount of abdominal discomfort after surgery.

When you're lying in bed after surgery, concentrating on deep, slow breathing is calming. It produces relaxation and improves the circulation and uptake of oxygen in your body — essential for healing. It also stimulates the flow of lymph — the body's defense system — against invading germs.

## Biofeedback

*Biofeedback* is a technique that gives us information about a function of the body that we're not usually aware of and over which we usually have no control. An example of one such function is the heart rate. With biofeedback, we can see how the mind affects the body. Before biofeedback was discovered, it was believed that certain of our body functions were completely automatic. Examples are the release of hormones, the narrowing and widening of blood vessels, the rate of the heart beat, peristalsis, the frequency of brainwaves. It's true that these work automatically; we wouldn't be able to think about much else if every moment we had to decide to make our hearts beat. But biofeedback has shown that we can have some voluntary control of these functions.

Biofeedback uses special equipment to measure functions such as your skin temperature, pulse rate, and brain wave frequency. The results of the measurements appear in a readout that you get to see and hear. The biofeedback subject sees or hears the readout. By trying to change the readout, you succeed in changing the bodily function being monitored. For example, by imagining that your hand is getting colder, you will lower the skin temperature and you'll be able to see the results on the screen.

Biofeedback is more than just an interesting experiment. It allows you to train yourself to take control over body functions that are normally completely automatic. After training, many patients are able to control these functions without using the machinery. Though not widely used now, biofeedback training could be useful for preoperative preparation. It could help to decrease tension in specific muscles. *Alpha wave brain training* (alpha is the general frequency of your brainwaves associated with the relaxed state) could be used before general anesthesia for relaxation, mental calmness and clarity. For skin grafts and muscle flaps, there could be temperature electrodes which patients could use to increase the blood supply to areas that need it. To reduce swelling, the patient using biofeedback could constrict the blood vessels. Biofeedback could also be used to constrict the blood flow to areas where surgical blood loss is extensive. These applications could be combined with hypnosis and visualization.

The information we get from biofeedback is encouraging to us because it shows us that we can change body functions we thought we couldn't control. If we know that we can do it, we *can* do it.

## Diet

Diet is an important part of health, but it probably won't be emphasized during your hospital stay unless you have a diet-specific disease like diabetes. You will have better surgical results (and better health in general) if you plan your diet carefully. You may have to consult a nutritionist or read books to get the right information. Keeping a healthy diet is more than just relying on federal guidelines for Recommended Daily Allowances (RDA) of vitamins and minerals. These recommended levels are minimal; they are designed only to protect the public from extreme deficiency diseases like scurvy and rickets which are not common today. If we want optimal health (and we do), our dietary needs will be more complicated.

While diet is important in maintaining optimal health, beware of anyone who claims to be able to cure anything and anyone through diet alone. Many foods have beneficial effects, but diet is only one aspect of keeping healthy.

Having access to foods you like in the hospital can have positive emotional and psychological effects on you. As a result, you may digest your food more efficiently. Even before you are allowed to eat again after surgery, just thinking about appetizing foods can stimulate your *peristalsis* (the contractions that help move the food through your body). You'll be less likely to vomit and will resume normal bowel functions more quickly.

## Exercise

You may not be able to exercise due to your condition. Other illnesses allow it. In any case, keep exercise from low to moderate before surgery. Running a marathon before your operation may boost your spirits in one way, but it can temporarily depress your immune system. Even if you can't exercise, you can still do controlled breathing exercises to work your diaphragm. If breathing is difficult for you, you may need a physical or respiratory therapist to give you special treatments. While lying in bed you can visualize your return to exercise, as well as continuing relaxation techniques. Hospitals have physical therapy departments that work hard to get you back into shape as soon as you are ready. Exercise stimulates the circulation of blood and lymph and produces endorphins for a feeling of well-being. If you feel worried or panicky about the surgery, it may help to go for a walk with a friend or family member.

It's certainly a temptation to cut out exercise altogether when approaching surgery, but it's a mistake. The key is the right level of exercise. Even if exercise must be curtailed, there will always be something you can do to get some of its benefits. For example, you can do stretching and breathing exercises.

## Music

Under general anesthesia you may not feel pain, and you may not remember anything, but you can hear. At this and all other times, sounds affect us profoundly. Our first sensations were probably hearing our mother's heart beating long before we were born. Sounds are vibrations we can sense, not only with our ears, but with our whole bodies. Sounds can be therapeutic to hear, and even more therapeutic to create ourselves.

When we sing, hum, or play an instrument, the body feels the vibrations more strongly than it does just listening. Of course, we may not be skilled at singing or playing an instrument. But we can still derive great benefit from the listening.

At Beth Israel Medical Center North in New York City
we have an organized program to give patients access to
music before surgery. Some patients bring in their own
tapes and others choose from our library. We often let the
patient bring the tape into the operating room to be played
through headphones during surgery — whether the patient
is awake or asleep. Many patients prefer baroque music
for its calming effects, but the choice is a highly individual
one. In almost all cases, however, some kind of music is
beneficial.

## Prayer and Religion

Metaphysics, sex, politics, and religion are best
avoided, we are told, in polite conversations. But without
question if you find comfort in spirituality, prayer, or
religion, it will help you when you go through surgery.
Parapsychologists believe in the human "spirit," a field of
energy that keeps the body and mind alive; it's the life
force. Its effects may be enhanced by peak experiences:
the times when everything works and we feel absolutely
wonderful. Many people who have been healed of diseases
that were considered incurable agree that they survived
because they were able to generate a feeling of uncondi-
tional love for themselves and others.

Most of us have some positive thoughts and images.
One of the most powerful is forgiveness. This doesn't
mean that it's bad to have healthy, normal anger in our
lives, but it does mean that we go to work on the resentment and ill will that may be hurting us. Healthy anger is
one of the natural ways we have of defending our boun-
daries. When expressed appropriately, it enhances our
self-esteem and immune responses. Unhealthy anger,
which is often unexpressed, can linger as prolonged
resentment. It can hamper our immune system's efforts to
fend off disease. It can also cause or contribute to depression.

Each person has his or her own personal way of dealing with these issues. Some turn to psychology, others to philosophy or religion. In all cases, there are many books and courses available. A healthy spirit can go far to compensate for the fact that your body may not be well.

Here's an active exercise you can do:

Before bedtime, just close your eyes and think about people who may have hurt you in the past. Imagine saying to that person, I forgive you and I release you. Then imagine that person saying to you, I forgive *you* and I release *you*. You can use the same technique in reverse if you're the one who feels in need of the forgiveness. With either technique, you bring in one person after another, until you resolve all the need for forgiveness.

You might have to repeat this exercise several times.

What if there is someone I can't forgive? Don't worry about it too much; at least try to release the pain that person caused you. Maybe you can go part way.

As you can see, most of the techniques in this chapter on *alternate* medicine aren't really alternate at all. They're out there for you to use together with techniques used in the hospital. The more you know, the better you will be able to use all the techniques and resources at your disposal.

# Thirteen

# How Much Do I Need to Know?

*Give me the liberty to know, to utter,
and to argue freely according to con-
science, above all liberties.*

Milton

**»** Emotional preparation is a fine thing, you say. And so is
being an informed medical consumer. But do I have to
know every detail about my medical problem? Must I
become familiar with every surgical nuance, every anesthetic technique? Isn't there any point at which I can relax,
lie back and trust skilled specialists to take care of me?
Don't they get paid exceptionally well to lift the burden of
anxiety from me?

There is no simple answer to any of these questions.
Your level of knowledge is more a matter of your personal
style. It's a matter of finding a middle ground that works
for you. What *is* clear is that the path of total ignorance
will not help you — it's likely to leave you sick and in pain.

Perhaps the better way to view the problem of how
much medical detail you should know is to see it in terms
of finding the right amount of anxiety. Anxiety? Isn't

anxiety always detrimental? No! A managed level of anxiety can lead to the most useful and positive state of mind that you can have for getting you through surgery. A *healthy level of anxiety* can spur a patient on to dealing with problems and fears.

Back in the 1950s, psychiatrist I.L. Janis analyzed levels of anxiety felt by patients facing surgery. Three main categories of surgical patient emerged. First there were those who were "scared stiff" of the surgery. These people seemed to resist every effort being made to calm them down. They are the ones who can make the jobs of hospital personnel very difficult indeed. At the other extreme were those who seemed to have a "piece of cake" attitude. These were people who refused to express any trepidation whatsoever. They showed little concern and left everything in the hands of their doctors and nurses. In the middle were people who were reasonably anxious about what was to happen to them. These people asked questions; they exhibited fear but seemed in control of their fear.

It was this middle group, it turned out, who did best after surgery. They had fewer complications, a lower level of pain complaint, and a better convalescence. They also tolerated hospital confinement and restrictions and their own temporary physical impairment with fewer complaints.

While it was expected that the "high anxiety" group would fare poorly in all these respects, the surprise finding was that the "piece of cake" group also did poorly. Many members of this group weren't truly attuned to their anxiety or else, in trying to be brave, made their anxiety worse. They seemed totally unprepared for their discomfort and were inconsolable. It's absolute nonsense to think that you can undergo surgery, no matter how routine or minor, without some anxiety. It's important to face the beast head on, to whittle anxiety down to manageable size.

This book is geared toward knowing more rather than less. How, then, to deal with the anxiety that knowing more can bring? Planning helps to sort all this out. Start your learning curve early, long before you check into the hospital. This way you will be able to digest your newly found knowledge in manageable chunks. You'll be able to use the knowledge you gain to create building blocks of emotional preparation. Flood the human psyche with too many things to understand all at once, and the result can be negative.

> A 1990 study was made of institutionalized psychiatric patients who underwent surgery for ailments not related to their psychological disability. It provided startling evidence of how a patient's emotional state can affect recovery from surgery. In this study of two hundred patients, those who were emotionally disabled had a postoperative complication rate *more than three times higher* than the non-institutionalized control group matched for age, sex and operation criteria. They remained in the hospital an average of three days longer.

How much you know or want to know is not just a theoretical question. More and more, patients are called upon to make informed choices. Your doctors might ask you to choose certain surgical or anesthetic options. You'll certainly have to become aware of how long your recovery period will be, how long you will be out of action, so you can arrange your work and family schedules.

In all but the most minor types of surgery something could go wrong. Your will should be in order before you go in. You may have considered creating a *living will*, indicating your views on receiving life support in extreme circumstances; the period before surgery is a good time to take care of this. The hospital will also want you to sign an informed consent before surgery. All of this paper work should be completed well before the day of surgery so you can resolve any anxiety it might cause. No one wants to be told about worst possible scenarios just before anesthesia, even if the scenarios are unlikely. Insist on getting all this out of the way ahead of time.

> *I believe that I should give the patient enough information about the plastic surgery I will be doing, but I skip the technical details. For instance, in a face lift, I emphasize to them that I do a face lift in two layers. I lift the expressive muscles in a separate procedure. I need to tell them where the scars are going to be. I don't want them to be surprised. But they don't need to know what kind of stitches I use. They need to know the basics about how the surgery is done, how long they will be in the operating room, and what the recovery period will be like.*
>
> Rosa Razaboni, MD

Starting with Hippocrates in ancient Greece, medicine has had a tradition of telling the patient as little as possible. The idea was to prevent anxiety. In this age of wide popular knowledge about medical problems and solutions, this "ignorance is bliss" philosophy has no place. The first item of intelligence you, the patient, must obtain is how much your doctor believes the patient should know. Each doctor deals with this troublesome question in his or her own way. If you want to know more than what you believe the doctor is telling you, you'll have to make that quite clear.

Our final response to the questions "How much do I need to know?" and "How much do I want to know?" is "As much as possible, but in the proper dosages." Ignorance can only hurt you. The trick is to take plenty of time learning what you have to learn. That way you can absorb the information. That way you can deal with the little anxieties as they come up. That way you keep the beast of fear in its rightful place—as a domesticated animal. For if you have any enemy when you go into the hospital, it's fear. As we shall see, you can't run from fear—it will find you. You've got to face it head on.

# Fourteen

# Fear

*Fear always springs from ignorance.*
Ralph Waldo Emerson

» Fear is a powerful negative force, even in day-to-day life. In the hospital, fear can be emotionally crippling and physically disabling. Fear, the uninvited guest in our hearts and minds, is Enemy Number One.

It doesn't take much imagination to find something to fear in a presurgical setting. What if something goes wrong? What if they find out something unpleasant when they open me up? What about the pain? Will I be disfigured by the surgery? When can I go home?

The question of surgical scars is an important one. Dr. Furlong has found in her practice that many patients are not aware of what their scars will look like, where they will be, how large they will be, and how long they will take to heal. The truth never hurts in this situation. "Often," she says, "patients have a positive reaction when they get to see their scars after surgery. It's a feeling of relief that helps them heal faster inside and out."

These are only a few examples of fears — we could list dozens, from the critical down to the trivial, but we don't want to frighten you unnecessarily. What is important is that the two great weapons against fear are both under your control. Knowledge is one of them. The other is attitude.

A brief word about knowledge. Why is knowledge *my* job? Don't I depend on the doctor (for all I am paying) to take care of the knowledge area? The answer is yes, but only for the *medical* knowledge. Even if the medical care is the world's finest, you can't assume medical personnel have the perspective to educate you away from your fears. They're focused, and that's good. They come in every day to do the same job, while you're in the hospital for only a brief period. That's why you're responsible for keeping informed.

If you keep a positive attitude, if you keep informed, you keep your level of emotional health high. Remember, your own judgment of yourself is important. It will affect the outcome of the surgery. If you believe you will have a smooth, rapid recovery, you probably will. If you let fear take over, you move in the other direction.

Most of the fears involved with surgery are reasonable, based on real risks. But if we don't watch our thought process, we can magnify these justifiable fears way out of proportion. We are afraid not only of the threat, *but of our own inability to deal with it*. It doesn't take much imagination to see how surgical/hospital fear can mushroom out of proportion when self-doubt comes into play.

Let's look at phobias—unreasonable fears—for a moment. Few people have phobias about horses, yet accidents involving horses hurt and kill hundreds of people every year. Snakes are widely feared, yet only a handful of people are hurt by snakes; few people ever *see* snakes in the wild. There's no rhyme or reason to it—the fear comes from within, not from a real threat. When dealing with a real threat, the strength to meet the challenge also comes from within. Since we deal with real, not imagined, threats in the hospital, knowledge does help to send the attitude in the right direction.

Unless you are a total failure at life, there must be something you do well—a job, a hobby, a sport. Be sure that people with wonderful capabilities in other areas may lack the confidence to do what you do. The skier who takes on every hill may turn into a jellyfish when asked to make a one-minute speech; the accomplished lecturer may be afraid to complain to a waiter about her soup being too cold; the ace waiter may be afraid to ask the bank for a loan. In each case self-image is high in at least one area, lacking in another. No one, however, can count on automatically discovering that he or she is superbly skilled in being a surgical patient. It takes a little thinking and a little work.

> Fear of surgical pain can itself make the pain worse. When you work on the fear you also work on the pain. The two areas are intimately related. It's essential to maintain and build your level of confidence so you can take both fear and pain in your stride.

Since you're already reading this book, you're on the right track to mastering your fears of surgery and the hospital experience. You're already educating yourself and learning to recognize and demand the finest level of care, particularly regarding pain management. You fully realize that the most dangerous part of going to the hospital is driving there in an automobile. In other words, you are *prepared*.

Certain mental techniques can build on your preparation to put your fear in its proper place.

- Concentrate on positive outcomes. All your thinking should be oriented toward successful surgery, minimal pain, effective healing. You've got to bat down and combat obtrusive thoughts that lead you away from positive outcomes. These thoughts can breed fear.

- Distract yourself with positive imagery. Bring into the hospital as many pleasant things as possible: a few favorite things from home, books, music you like and, by all means, your teddy bear (the hospital gift shop will be happy to sell you a bear if you don't already own one).

- Relax. Relaxation means different things to different people. For some, it may mean lots of activity, for others, deep breathing. In any case, don't just lie there worrying. Keep yourself occupied in ways that build you. We'll take you through some relaxation procedures later on.

- Family and friends can help you, but try to surround yourself with those who consistently build you up. Avoid the ones who drain you.

What you cannot and must not do is ignore the fear factor. You are human, and you have the possibility of fear. Scientists have theorized that some people, either because of their genetic background or due to the way they were raised, are more emotionally sensitive and prone to fear than others. For our purposes, this means that these people must just work a little harder. For anybody, if you do nothing, fear will find you. Every aspect of your surgical experience will suffer.

The key to dealing with fear is to get yourself moving in the right direction, not to wipe out fear entirely. It's natural to be afraid. Some anxiety can be helpful. If you face your fear instead of burying it, you keep it from getting out of control.

# Fifteen

# How Can I Prepare?

*Things done well and with a care,*
*exempt themselves from fear.*
William Shakespeare

» Why do I have to prepare myself for surgery? you might ask. Don't I pay good money so others can see to everything for me? For that matter, I'm going to be "out cold" while the main action is going on. I'm going to be sedated before and after. What's the fuss?

This entire book is about preparation for surgery. Without preparation we are prey to discomfort, uncertainty, and mind-numbing fear. We're liable to spend a longer time in the hospital and to recover much more slowly once we get home. The strain on our family and friends will be greater. Insurance or no, we might even spend more money. Preparation is key.

How do you prepare when there is so much to do? Step-by-step. Methodically. By learning. By communicating. By controlling your environment at critical periods. By training your subconscious mind.

And lest we forget, a little self-indulgence goes a long way. Treat yourself well before going into the hospital. Get a massage, take a few extra days off from work, read a book, have an ice cream cone.

We've broken down the preparation and planning steps into seven basic areas involving knowledge, communication, and environment.

## Knowledge — Learning What You Need to Know

- **Preparation Area One: Knowledge From Outside.** You'll want to collect as much medical information as you can in three basic areas. The *first* involves the general medical area: what was wrong with you in the first place; why you need surgery to correct the problem. The *second* involves knowledge about how the surgery will be done and how long the healing process will take. The *third* involves anesthesia and pain control questions.

- **Preparation Area Two: Knowledge of the Inside.** You'll want to know as much as possible about yourself and how you react to medical treatment. Were you hospitalized as a child; did you have surgery then? Can you remember problems with pain control or fear of pain? If you are undergoing cosmetic surgery, have you made sure your expectations are realistic? How do you assess your general level of health and fitness? What about your emotional state; is this surgery coming at a good time in your life? Do you see the surgery as a formative life experience or as a threat? It pays to have a long talk with yourself on these matters, to keep a journal, to write things down. Assuming you've already written down practical questions for your doctor, the journal also gives you a place to record your emotional needs and reactions. It allows you to express your feelings instead of holding them in. It helps you to clarify your thoughts.

> If you're feeling very low about yourself and nothing seems to be going right, take a chair and sit in front of a mirror. Talk to that worried person. Ask your mirror image to unburden its heart. After the out-pouring of worries and tears, you will start to see some smiles.

## Communication — Making Your Needs and Desires Known

- **Preparation Area Three: Communication With Medical People.** Make a list of all medical and hospital personnel you'll be coming into contact with: your family doctor, the surgeon, the anesthesiologist, the nurses, perhaps a counselor or psychotherapist. Write down questions you wish to ask about matters that concern you. Rework and revise the list, making it as clear and concise as possible. Make sure these questions get asked and answered to your satisfaction. Are there special things the doctors and nurses should know about you? If your vision, speech, or hearing is impaired, it may have a severe impact on your ability to communicate your needs. The medical team will need to work with you to create ways of communicating.

- **Preparation Area Four: Communication With Yourself.** Again, a long talk with yourself. Like any life experience that isn't routine (graduation, getting a new job, getting married, becoming a parent, losing a loved one), going to the hospital should be a chance to reflect on your life, its direction and needs. Ask yourself probing questions and give yourself well-thought-out answers. Why not make this break in your life as formative as possible?

- **Preparation Area Five: Communication With Family and Friends.** Much of the communication you have with family and friends is implicit. You don't spell everything out because you don't have to. But when dealing with hospitalization and surgery, you must be very careful to make your needs known and to get people who care about you as involved as possible. Don't assume *they* know what you know or feel what you feel. Ask them for help in so many words. And don't assume that *you* know what you need either. Taking care of some of your own needs may have become such an ingrained habit that you lack the perspective to recognize what they are.

## Environment — Creating a Positive Atmosphere

- **Preparation Area Six: The Physical Environment.** Plan for your own comfort both in the hospital and while recuperating at home. Make sure you have some familiar personal things in your hospital room. If, for example, you will not be on a restricted diet, find out if alternates to hospital food are available (like outside delivery). You might want to arrange to have a VCR or personal stereo in your room. You'll have more control over what you watch or listen to than if you just have a TV or radio — relaxation, health, humorous or self-developmental material, for example. If friends and family will be visiting you, it may be wise to familiarize yourself with public transportation schedules, parking restrictions in the area, local restaurants and other details. A blanket or quilt, your own pillow, or a teddy bear will round out the environment. Don't leave your comfort to chance.

- **Preparation Area Seven: The Mental Environment.** A good physical environment has a positive effect on the mental environment of course, but the mental environment is an area in itself. If music inspires or relaxes you, make sure you have access to it. If you like to read, choose your reading matter with care so it's uplifting and enjoyable rather than just time-consuming. The hospital is an excellent place to work with personal growth and self-developmental materials. Specific mind/body pain prevention and healing techniques like the use of suggestion tapes before, during, and after general anesthesia, are discussed throughout this book. Active techniques oriented toward creating a positive mind-set will yield the best results. But start at home, sometime before you enter the hospital.

> Your own preparation for surgery should be extensive. Just as the anesthesiologist checks out critical machinery, it's up to you to make sure your personal support network is in place and that you have the best level of knowledge possible about the procedures you will be going through. The end result will be optimum medical care, meaningful pain control and effective healing.

## The Preoperative Visit

Your final meeting with the anesthesiologist will probably be at the preoperative visit (pre-op in hospital speak). Expect one. Insist on one. The visit is a two-way street. The anesthesiologist needs to learn as much as possible about you. It's your turn to ask final questions — even to discuss your fears. This is no place to be afraid of appearing ignorant or foolish. You need to know many things. The magic word is *ASK.*

Dr. Egbert did a controlled study finding that patients who received supportive preoperative visits had better results, less pain, and faster healing than other patients whose interviews were perfunctory. The state-of-the-art anesthesiologist follows this philosophy. Nevertheless, not all patients get the opportunity to have a pre-op visit. Many surgical situations have time constraints, especially if you don't sleep at the hospital the night before. The pre-op visit should be an extra reassurance, but even without it you should see to it that you are fully prepared and attuned to your own special needs.

## Self-Medication

A word on self-medication is in order here, since it's a serious problem. A 1992 study of ambulatory surgical patients showed that over a quarter of them—without telling their doctors—took some kind of medication themselves because of their fear of surgical and postsurgical pain. The premedication ranged from sleeping pills and alcohol to cocaine to marijuana. Obviously, a good proportion of surgical patients have real fears of undergoing unnecessary pain due to undermedication, so much so that they risked dangerous complications by secretly medicating themselves. The advisable course is to coordinate all medication with the physicians responsible for pain control. Self-controlled *emotional* preparation is by far the safest and most effective patient strategy.

If you are on medication you might be told by the admitting office or the surgeon not to take anything by mouth for the twelve hours or more before surgery. If you think you will need the medication—say for pain control—don't be shy about asking the anesthesiologist if you can take the medication anyhow. Most anesthesiologists will encourage you to continue your medication. More and more, patients are also being allowed clear liquids up to four hours before surgery. One warning: if you take a strong sedative before coming to the hospital and have not yet signed your consent for surgery, your operation may be canceled. Sign the consent beforehand.

# Sixteen

# How Can Other People Help Me?

*As the yellow gold is tried in fire, so the faith of friendship must be seen in adversity.*

**Ovid**

» Surgery is a time in your life when you most need the support of your family, friends, and co-workers. They care a great deal about you. They really want to help you, but you have to ask them and guide them.

Sure, you're tough. Other people don't feel your pain or worry your worries. You could "go it alone" if you had to. But you don't have to. When people really care about each other, problems — even crises — can and should bring them closer together. You and the people close to you end up with more after the crisis passes than you had before.

The first step is getting friends and family involved. Rather than gripe and complain to them, let them know exactly what kind of surgery you will be going through. What are the risks? How long will the healing process take? Show them where you are brave and where you might chicken out.

At Beth Israel Medical Center North in New York City, where Dr. Furlong practices, family and friends are made more an integral part of the patient's surgical experience. The hospital is allowing supporters to wait with the patient before surgery. Volunteers are there to pass messages from the patient in the recovery room to the relatives and friends waiting elsewhere. Some rooms are equipped to allow guests to stay overnight. As Dr. Furlong stresses, bringing in people close to the patient is better medicine than giving them a shot. When she sees somebody holding the patient's hand, she knows they're going to do well. The conventional wisdom sees outsiders as being in the way, but their love and support are just as healing as the doctor's technical expertise.

Very often, surprisingly, it's the patient worrying about the visitor, rather than the other way around. Dr. Furlong has seen many a patient relax when she told them that their mother in the waiting room was doing fine.

The next step is cementing networks of emotional support. Communicate your needs and listen to what your friends and family have to say. The fears and concerns of others are often very useful when you need to pinpoint your own. Remember, people close to you may have their own worries and fears about you. Your personal fear control program should include them. Studies have shown that family caregivers to people with difficult illnesses often suffer both mentally and physically as a result. Your task is to bring them in to help, without making them do the worrying for you. Together, if you work in the same direction, you both can keep the fear under control.

Emotional support is important, but so is advocacy. At least one friend or family member should be there to act as your advocate in case you can't speak for yourself. For example, you might be in pain after surgery but too sedated to properly ask for appropriate medication. The friend should either know as much as you know or be instructed to ask for certain specific medical care for you at certain critical times. Include the friend in the planning process. A situation to be avoided is one where more than one friend or family member fights to be the patient's advocate. With the emotional burden this creates, often the message doesn't get through very clearly to the health personnel involved.

> When you have a medical prob-
> lem — especially if it's a complicated
> one — you might be tempted to
> "tough it out" by going it alone.
> Avoid this temptation. Now is when
> you need familiar faces around you
> to give you support.

Yes, asking for help from friends and family members can be touchy. But think of this — most people really like to help others if they believe their help will be honestly appreciated. If you learn to really communicate with people who care about you, you don't have to make them feel guilty. Your relationship with some friends and family members may be difficult. But direct, clear communication and an honest open request for help and involvement is always the best course.

Co-workers and people you deal with but are not very close with can still give you necessary support through your surgery and recovery. Whatever your position — boss or subordinate — you must make sure your co-workers, employees, or clients have at least a rough idea of how long you will be out of action. Be realistic; don't have them expecting you back at work too early. If your medical problem is not serious, make good and sure they know that. If you don't, they will begin to entertain the notion that they could get along without you. If it *is* serious, how much you tell them depends on the circumstances and on individual relationships. If you work with people every day, a telephone progress report once or twice while you're away is both a courtesy and a minimal involvement tool.

The question of pets is an important one. Many people are extremely attached to their pets (or to animals in general) and get great emotional support from their pets. But few hospitals allow pets (we don't know of any). A photo of the pet can be surprisingly uplifting, however. One of Dr. Furlong's patients had nearly died from cardiac arrest in a previous surgery and was in a state of panic. In trying to calm the patient down, the subject of pets came up. Fortunately Dr. Furlong had a photo of Ilkley, her Yorkshire terrier. The patient looked at the photo of this adorable dog several times before surgery. Ilkley's sweet little face was the last thing she remembered before losing consciousness. The photo was the first thing she asked for when she woke in the recovery room. "It may seem silly, but your dog's photograph saved my life," the patient said.

# Seventeen

# Great Expectations: The Ideal Scenario

*The talent of success is nothing more than doing what you can do well.*

Longfellow

» The day for your surgery arrives, and everything is going to go right. Your mental and emotional houses are in order. You have communicated your needs to the people who will be treating you, to your family and friends, to yourself. You have made arrangements for an optimum environment for both body and mind. So you can relax now. Right?

Right. You expected us to say *Wrong*, didn't you? But, the fact is, all the work and preparation has just one goal, to *allow* you to relax, to be confident, to be free from worry and fear.

The process of things going right has many individual steps. Let's recount them.

- You have learned as much as possible about your medical problem and how it's to be alleviated through surgery. You have considered going for a second opinion, and are satisfied that you have made the right decision about having surgery.

- You have chosen your surgeon with some care. You've looked to see that the surgeon uses modern techniques that can cause you less pain and hasten your healing process.
- You have done basic consumer research on the hospital where you will be having the surgery. You have chosen a hospital with a pain control service or with a history of effective pain control work.
- You have learned as much as possible about how the surgical technique will work.
- You have learned as much as possible about the different alternatives for anesthesia and pain control.
- You understand from your anesthesiologist what procedures will be used and what kind of anesthesia you will be having.
- You have given your anesthesiologist information about your physical condition, possible drug reactions, and allergies.
- You have had a long talk with yourself to try to understand what your fears and worries are. You begin to keep a journal of your thoughts.
- You have made a thorough personal analysis of your history of dealing with various kinds of pain and how you handled and reacted to the pain.
- You have made a personal assessment of your general level of health and fitness so your healing expectations can be realistic.
- You begin the process of involving family, friends and co-workers in your hospitalization in a responsible, meaningful, well-managed way to benefit all concerned.
- You communicate your needs to appropriate medical personnel, especially the anesthesia personnel responsible for pain control. You also question them about

possible prejudices against narcotic use, in order to avoid possible undermedication.

- If your hearing or speech is impaired, if you can't see without your glasses on, you've let your medical team and your friends know, so that alternate means of communication have been worked out (or you've kept your glasses or hearing aid with you).

> Since you've remained well informed through every phase of the surgical process, and since you've insisted on your right to proper medical care and pain control, everything is going swimmingly. They'll close your incision, and you'll be out of the hospital in no time.

- You talk with the nurses and admissions people about your environmental needs while in the hospital — extra blankets, for example.

- You write down what your environmental needs are, so that they can best be filled.

- You prepare your mental environment by choosing appropriate self-developmental or inspirational materials (books, audio cassettes and music) to be at hand during your hospitalization.

- You practice stress-reducing and fear-reducing techniques prior to surgery.

- You choose or create an audiotape with positive healing or developmental suggestions to be played back or read to you during general anesthesia and surgery.

- You ask the surgeon or anesthesiologist to say only positive things to you while you're under anesthesia and to avoid certain conversational topics.
- You develop a clear plan of what you'll be doing after surgery, from the recovery room to your return to home, work, and normal activities.
- After surgery, either you, a friend, or a relative pays attention to the level of pain medication you're being given, making sure that it's given to you in proper dosages and at proper intervals.
- After surgery, you continue working with self-developmental materials and stress and fear-reducing techniques.
- After surgery, both in the hospital and during the first few days or weeks at home, you continue to monitor your environment to make sure it's both physically and mentally conducive to healing.
- You obey your doctor's orders about how soon you can go back to normal activities, especially work or physical exercise. You also listen to your body if it tells you not to rush things.
- You close the door on your surgical experience, as whole as you were before. Perhaps the experience has even given you time to think, reflect, and grow as a human being.

# Eighteen

# The Less Than Ideal Scenario

*A wise man should consider that health is the greatest of human blessings, and learn how by his own thought to derive benefit from his illnesses.*

Hippocrates

Since we've already gone over what you can do to make your surgery a ringing success, it may be useful to discuss a case where the results were not that good. We're not assuming technically poor results here, only that the experience will be much more worrisome, more painful, and filled with fear and unknowing. You'll probably be in the hospital longer, and you may undergo significant psychological damage.

What do you have to do to achieve such an undesirable result? Well, no checklist is in order here. The answer to that question is plain and simple. Nothing!

- If you do nothing, other people will decide when you are feeling pain and how much medication you need. You'll be the last person consulted.

- If you do nothing, you will be fair game to every fear your imagination can manufacture.

- If you do nothing, you will be constantly in the dark about what is happening to you. And ignorance is not bliss.

- If you do nothing, you will be leaving up to chance whether state-of-the-art surgical and pain control procedures will be available, or if they will be used if available.

- If you do nothing, you run a greater risk of drug reactions and side effects. (Often both you and your doctors will have to do some intelligent digging into your medical history to get the whole picture.)

- If you do nothing, all the negative environmental stimuli, like stray talk, will enter your brain without any filter or buffer at the brain's most sensitive time.

> Things will not go well for you in a surgical setting if you lie back and expect all the thinking and deciding to be done for you. No one else can feel your pain. No matter how skilled the doctors and nurses are, they don't have the telepathic ability to guess your exact needs and concerns.

- If you do nothing, you will have no control over the gates that regulate the transmission of pain signals. You will "learn" pain, "remember" pain, "re-create" and echo pain needlessly.

- If you do nothing, your time in the hospital and during recovery will drag, one meaningless hour following another, time not only wasted, but damaging to your well-being.

- If you do nothing, you will lose valuable opportunities to involve people close to you in an important experience in your life.

- If you do nothing and things go wrong, your family may not be able to decide on your treatment in the absence of specific instructions or a living will.

- If you do nothing, you undergo stress and damage your general health.

- If you do nothing, your healing process is haphazard. In many areas of your health, it may well be incomplete.

- If you do nothing, you never really close the door on your negative health experience. Emotionally, nothing is truly resolved.

We've just painted a depressing scenario. Unfortunately, it's also a common scenario. But this is not the way *you* will approach your surgical experience. You're a vital, positive person with an indomitable will to be healthy, to live your life to the fullest. You know what to do to make the surgical process a positive one. You do it.

# Nineteen

# People Used to Laugh at Lamaze

*To live a single day and hear a good teaching is better than to live a hundred years without knowing such teaching.*

Buddha

» Lamaze and other "natural" childbirth techniques used to be on the fringe—now they are mainstream. In the same way, techniques to conquer chronic and surgical pain are becoming better known and more widely accepted. It's only a matter of time before these techniques become part of standardized, well-tested programs. Once this happens, surgical patients and chronic pain sufferers will have greater access in their communities to expert advice on controlling pain.

But advice is not the only key to the problem. Involvement and training of the people who actually feel the pain are even more important. And that's what the future holds. The public demands much more from the healing professions than it did a generation ago. From far and wide the cry has been heard—I will not accept unnecessary pain.

One of the problems with pain is that it can't be seen, felt, or even measured by the person not suffering from it. In terms of research, pain is not "sexy." It's much easier for a researcher to do research on a rare disease that offers tangible results than to work on alleviating pain (where the only reward may be the patient's eternal gratitude). In reality, pain is suffered so widely, so unnecessarily, that it insists on remaining a major public health issue.

> Both surgical and chronic pain are major problems among the population as a whole. Consciousness of modern solutions to pain control, particularly involving the mind/body connection, is rising. It's only a matter of time before the public at large becomes knowledgeable about and sensitive to effective pain control teachings.

As we have seen, pain can damage and kill. When a person who is in danger of pain learns to keep the pain at bay, that person achieves a degree of freedom—a real self-control. We all want and need to know that we do have control over our bodies, that doctors don't know everything about our reactions and feelings.

As bright minds strive to solve the difficult healthcare problems the United States faces, the brightest must come again and again to the issue of wellness, to quality of life. Wellness does involve doctors, but even more it involves teachers, social workers, community organizations, and schools. Widespread teaching about pain control and alleviation is an important part of wellness.

People train for natural childbirth for many weeks in every community now, though the idea was ridiculed not a generation ago. The many millions of anesthetic procedures performed annually far outnumber the number of childbirths. There is so much that the pain sufferer can do — from heightened awareness to breathing exercises to learning to deal with fear and stress — that doctors simply don't have the time to teach on a last-minute basis. Training programs therefore make good sense. We'll be seeing a lot more of them in the coming years.

# Twenty

# Anesthesia in Childbirth

*Why is it that we rejoice at a birth? It is because we are not the person involved.*

Mark Twain

» Mark Twain was a little too cynical. Of course we should rejoice at the birth of a baby. But going through labor is not always a picnic. Childbirth is an area where the public's knowledge of anesthesia and pain control technique is at its highest. More and more, the patients — child-bearing women — are becoming aware and involved in medical decision making.

Barring an emergency, the anesthesiologist will review your medical chart and confer with your obstetrician. The anesthesiologist will be particularly careful to spot any incidence of hypertension or diabetes, two major areas where complications can arise due to childbirth. As with any administration of anesthesia, it's important to keep track of when you had your last meal. It's best to have as empty a stomach as possible, but with childbirth, it's not always possible to know in advance when that last meal should occur.

"Natural" childbirth has many adherents. The theory behind it is that fear of pain in childbirth makes the mother tense. The fear and tension make the process more difficult and more painful. As a result, many women go to classes that prepare them to have their babies in as relaxed a way as possible. Often the father will take part. The Lamaze method, the Leboyer technique, and the Bradley method are three popular techniques. By using these methods, millions of women have given birth, with a reduced need for analgesia and anesthesia. Some women even dispense with pain-killing medication altogether. Nurse/midwife Diane Moore. cautions expectant parents to be sure to use an accredited course and to avoid classes with more than ten couples; individual attention is very important.

The question of natural childbirth is a controversial one. Only you can decide which way to go. Bear in mind, however, that unnecessary pain helps no one. Anesthesia during labor involves balancing the mother's need for pain control with the need to protect the newborn infant from possible harm due to the anesthesia. The balance is delicate. While "natural" childbirth is a fine idea, it's certainly not appropriate when the woman is contemplating thirty hours of labor. Perhaps the best advice would be to train for and plan for "natural" childbirth if possible, but to learn about anesthesia anyway and be ready for it just in case the going gets rough. The best advice: be prepared both mentally and physically. Go through a course and learn everything you can. The anesthesia alone can't take care of all your pain. Some kind of relaxation exercise is important, even if "natural" childbirth isn't for you.

*There is no better delivery than a drug free delivery. It should be as natural as possible but this does not mean the mother has to be a hero. If she has severe pain a mild sedative can be given in the early stages of labor; sometimes this even helps to dilate the cervix (the opening of the uterus the baby will eventually emerge from). The more education and training about labor and childbirth the mother has, the less pain and distress she will suffer whether or not she has totally natural or epidural assisted birth and labor. Classes start in the last three months of pregnancy and often the nurse in the classroom may be one of the nurses present at delivery.*

Richard Scuderi, MD,
Lenox Hill Hospital
New York

*Epidural* and *spinal* anesthesia are commonly used in obstetrics. Each involves an injection in the spinal area. Spinals can lead to a "spinal headache" in about five percent of cases, while epidurals, which involve higher doses of drugs, can on rare occasions cause toxicity problems. Nevertheless, spinals and epidurals are preferred over general anesthesia for the important reason that a general anesthetic is more likely to cross the placenta and enter the baby's bloodstream. The epidural or spinal will rarely effect the baby unless the mother's blood pressure falls enough to affect blood flow to the baby. This side effect is not truly significant because the anesthesiologist, who is right by your side monitoring vital signs throughout labor, would immediately administer fluids and medications to boost blood circulation. The mother's blood pressure is also affected by the pressure of the uterus on the major blood vessels in the mother's abdomen. The anesthesiologist will have the mother avoid lying flat on her back, in order to reduce that pressure.

Since epidurals allow the woman in labor to hold normally uncomfortable positions for long periods of time, however, there is a chance of some degree of inadvertent back injury.

One in four childbirths in America is now a cesarian, and these, too, are usually done under an epidural or spinal unless there is an emergency. In an emergency, general anesthesia is preferred because it takes less time. Since the general is very light (to protect the infant), the mother may remain awake, although very drowsy. If this is explained beforehand, most mothers don't experience any trauma from being aware.

One of the enticements of "natural" childbirth is the idea of being awake during the process and welcoming and holding your baby after birth. With epidurals and spinals, it's your option. If the process makes you squeamish, ask for sedation.

Many couples believe that the father should be in the room with the mother for most or all of the process. That's all right, as long as the staff doesn't have to neglect the mother to prevent the father from fainting, or stop their work to answer his questions. If the father is queasy, he shouldn't be pressured to remain in the room. Having him sit rather than stand can prevent most faintness. But unless these problems occur, the father's presence is important. The staff has a responsibility to help him relax. Not only can the father's presence be a comfort to the mother, but the childbirth itself is an event both parents want and need to share.

# Twenty-One

# Anesthesia for Children

*Tis the eye of childhood that fears a painted devil.*

**Shakespeare**

» Children undergoing surgery have special medical and emotional needs. It has been said that when one family member is sick it affects the whole family. Nothing could be truer in the case of a sick child, especially when the illness is serious. The child is too young to use many of the techniques we recommend. The parents need to keep a positive attitude while allowing the child to express his or her fears or discomforts. Many adults remember being taken to the hospital as children for tonsillectomies, being told nothing more than that they were going to have ice cream, then waking up with pain, nausea, vomiting — and a hatred of the adults who lied to them. This simply will not do today.

The keyword in pediatric pain, whether chronic or surgical, is *undermedication*. There are three reasons for this. First, children, especially infants, are thought to be neurologically immature, hence less sensitive to pain.

Second, physicians fear that children can have special sensitivities to many anesthetics, and so they give them less rather than more. Third, and very important, children often have difficulty expressing their needs for pain medication, especially if they have not yet learned to speak.

With any pain management procedure that requires patient participation, feedback, and cooperation, children must be treated with special sensitivity. The more experienced the practitioner is in working with children, the better.

> *The effect of medication on children is very different from the effect on adults. The dosage usually used on children is generally based on the child's weight and body configuration. In my experience it doesn't necessarily stand up to the real pain control needs. I do think that basically we have a tendency out of fear to undermedicate. Using the child's weight as a guide to dosage doesn't take psychological and other factors that can increase or diminish pain into consideration.*
>
> Morrison S. Levbarg, MD, FAAP
> Medical Director
> Shield Institute, New York City

It's impossible, for example, to know whether a newborn is crying our of fear, discomfort, or pain. In addition, newborns may be hypersensitive to narcotics; careful respiratory monitoring will be necessary. Doctors are coming to realize that infants need to be properly medicated, then carefully monitored for side effects. Undermedication is simply not an acceptable alternative. For an infant or young child, the pain and stress that result from undermedication must be terrifying.

We've already seen how grown-up patients under general anesthesia can suffer damage from disturbing stimuli that reach the brain, despite general anesthesia. The patient lies still, seemingly unconscious; the surgeon can operate without considering the patient's pain; yet the damage is done. An infant or young child is in a similar situation. The child won't or can't complain. Everything seems all right to the surgeon. Yet the situation may be far from rosy. Being in the hospital itself may be traumatic for the child. Traumatic pain, stress, and fear during surgery can do far-reaching emotional damage. As we have seen, unnecessary pain during surgery can lead to worsening postsurgical pain, slower healing, and a longer stay in the hospital.

> Anesthesia and pain control for children have their own particular set of problems. The worst problem is that children often can't express or describe their pain and discomfort; even if they can speak, they may be subject to fear, inhibition, or embarrassment. It takes special communication skills among the adults involved to make sure children receive appropriate pain relief.

Using a hospital with an organized pain management service is especially important when children are involved. Many of these services have great expertise on chronic pain in children, such as that suffered by cancer patients. If your hospital has such a service, you stand a greater chance of finding the best combination of sensitivity and modern medical resources for the control of your child's physical pain and emotional stress. A useful pediatric pain measurement scale consists of drawings of faces ranging from smiling to frowning to crying. The child circles the appropriate face. Drawing is a known, effective means for children to express some of their needs. They should have paper, pencils, and crayons handy.

As to the anesthetics and sedatives themselves, these can often be administered to children orally or by skin patches, so as to avoid scary injections.

Another question is whether the parent should be present in the operating room with the child. Some doctors say it may make the child more nervous. Others believe that it only makes the doctor much more nervous. Even if the parents are not in the operating room, they should remain with the child at least until the child is sedated.

There are many techniques that work to put children at ease. In all cases the child should bring one or two favorite toys, perhaps a well-loved blanket. Most hospitals will let a child bring a toy to the operating room. At Memorial Hospital in New York City, you can arrange for a clown from the Big Apple Circus to wheel your child to the operating room. In some hospitals the parents can stay overnight with the children. You may also be able to prepare your child for hospitalization by visiting the hospital beforehand with the child, taking a tour of the equipment, meeting some of the staff. If you are active in your community, you may want to work to encourage hospitals to provide organized educational tours for children.

Dr. Beth Brodman, a pediatric anesthesiologist at Montefiore Hospital in New York, encourages one parent to come into the operating room for the induction of anesthesia. The parent dresses in a "rabbit suit," a paper-jumpsuit, including mask and hat. The parent might hold the child and help put on the face mask. The child goes to sleep breathing the anesthetic gases. The parent then leaves so Dr. Brodman can get on with the anesthesia and preparation for surgery. Once the child is asleep, the presence of a parent can be quite distracting to both anesthesiologist and surgeon. The main goal is for the parent to be present until the child goes to sleep. If the child is already asleep, the parent's presence isn't necessary.

Older children should be given some knowledge of what will be happening to them. It's a good idea that they be made to realize they will feel some discomfort after the surgery and that they'll get some medicine to help them feel better.

All children have vivid imaginations. We've seen the negative side of this, but there's also a positive side. It's easy to distract a child from pain, with stories. Some children can even be taught to control their pain by using imaginary switches. Children are particularly amenable to hypnosis. While they have special needs in surgery, there are many resources for meeting those needs.

# Twenty-Two

# Side Effects

*Some remedies are worse than the disease.*

Publilius Syrus

» The medications used in modern-day anesthesia are remarkably safe, and dangerous reactions to them are extremely rare. But we all react differently to medication. Some patients have multiple side effects while others have none.

What do we mean by side effects? A side effect is something the drug or procedure does that is extra to the desired effect. It's often unwanted. For example, morphine is an excellent pain reliever, but it can cause nausea and vomiting in some patients, a slowdown in breathing in others. While not every patient suffers from these side effects, they are frequent enough to be considered "normal." If you have unwanted effects, you and your doctor might choose a substitute drug, or you may want to use additional medications to combat or reverse the unwanted effects.

The most common side effects of anesthesia are nausea, sleepiness, dizziness, forgetfulness, inability to concentrate, and, less commonly, sore throat and difficulty in passing urine — all lasting from a few hours to a few days after surgery. Patients sometimes complain about having a funny taste or dryness in their mouths.

Regional (spinal or epidural) anesthesia can also lead to headaches. The headaches aren't dangerous, but they can be annoying when the patient needs to rest and recuperate. The use of morphine or other narcotics for postoperative pain relief administered through the epidural or spinal route can sometimes have side effects. These include a slowing of the breathing rate, itching and problems passing urine. Effective treatments are available for all these side effects.

> Neither you nor your anesthesiologist has any control over whether medications give you side effects. The more both of you learn about how you react to medications, the better.

As with any medical treatment that involves drugs, your personal medical history is important. New medications are being developed to get better anesthetic effects with fewer side effects. If you have either a history of side effects from particular anesthetics or a history of allergy, it's important to tell the anesthesiologist. That way you both can make special plans to avoid the offending agents.

Many people expect nausea after anesthesia. This is less and less of a concern, now that ether is no longer used. Ether caused a good deal of nausea and vomiting. Even though modern agents cause much less nausea and vomiting, the reputation has stuck. It's important to be aware of this, because an expectation of nausea can increase the likelihood of nausea coming on.

The mind has a definite effect on the stomach and digestive system. Try this experiment. Close your eyes. Imagine a big bowl of lemons. Feel the waxiness of the skin. Smell the subtle lemon smell. Pick up one of the lemons in one hand. In your other hand take a sharp knife. Cut the lemon lengthwise. Cut it again. Now take a big bite out of the lemon wedge.

You probably felt a lot of saliva in your mouth. Your mouth may have puckered up. You might even feel it in your stomach. But it was an imaginary lemon! Your stomach is a sensitive emotional barometer.

How do we get our stomachs to behave after anesthesia? One very powerful technique to get the *peristalsis* (the normal contractions of the stomach and intestines) going correctly again is to imagine your favorite food. This will get your stomach grumbling and growling and on its way to working the way it should.

But what about the people who say, "I get sick as a dog every time I get anesthesia." Look at it this way, this means that you are having *a very healthy reaction*. The body has built-in protective mechanisms. If you ate poison, immediately your brain would send a message to your stomach to remove the poison. The body might interpret the presence of anesthesia in the system as an unwanted substance. It isn't necessary to vomit, because your lungs, kidneys, and liver do a great job in removing all these substances. Merely telling your brain not to send the message to vomit...works.

Family history is especially important in the case of certain rare complications, such as malignant hyperthermia or the inability to metabolize the muscle relaxant succinylcholine. But it's a mistake to spend too much of your time and energy looking into one-in-a-million possibilities. If a rare dangerous reaction to anesthesia ran in your family, you would likely know about it. Anesthesia is extremely safe.

It's not possible here to cover every side effect and adverse drug reaction. But ask your anesthesiologist how much you need to know about the possible side effects of the specific agents and techniques the doctor recommends. Some people become more anxious with knowledge, some people less.

Remember, however, that dealing with side effects is in the mainstream of an anesthesiologist's practice. As we have discussed, you can also use your own techniques to deal with side effects such as nausea. Communicate with your doctors and nurses. They can treat your side effects, when possible, and give you reassurance when treatment isn't necessary.

# Twenty-Three

# Safety

*As soon as there is life there is danger.*
Emerson

» We've already mentioned that going under anesthesia is far safer than driving to the hospital. Let's expand on this. It's also much safer than *walking* to the hospital. According to the National Safety Council, twenty-two hundred pedestrians were struck down and killed on rural roads in one recent year. During the same period, about one hundred and fifty anesthesia-related deaths occurred. Anesthesia is given by doctors, nurse anesthetists, or dentists about 30 million times a year. Taking walks down country roads is also popular, yet twenty times more dangerous. Walking in the city is something else again. Even worse is driving a car. Automobile accidents kill one in fifty Americans.

Human beings react in complex ways when put under anesthesia, no matter how simple the surgery. Anesthesia uses highly sophisticated equipment and requires skilled, resourceful personnel. Most of the safety work is done before, not during, surgery. Stringent Food and Drug Administration (FDA) guidelines govern how anesthesia machines are manufactured, monitored, and serviced. Equally strict guidelines affect how they are used. The same kind of attention ensures that drugs used in anesthesia are safe, effective, and appropriate. At each critical juncture, set training and operating routines have been promulgated. They are adhered to.

For example, the FDA spells out procedures for checking anesthesia equipment right before use. The guidelines have been put into effect with great success. The FDA has also sponsored surveys which investigate the age and condition of anesthesia machines in hospitals all across the country. In cooperation with the Anesthesia Patient Safety Foundation, drug companies, and equipment manufacturers, the FDA has developed extensive educational programs. These programs make sure that knowledge about state-of-the-art safety equipment and techniques reaches anesthesia departments everywhere in the U.S. The Anesthesia Patient Safety Foundation reports that, from the viewpoint of lawyers and insurance professionals, anesthesia is a decidedly low-risk specialty.

> **Modern anesthesia is exceptionally safe — and getting safer!**

The question of side effects aside, most problems that do occur in anesthesia have to do with human error rather than equipment failure. Equipment that is properly maintained and checked will be effective if properly used. The anesthesiologist knows what to do when something goes wrong with equipment before or during surgery. A properly run anesthesia department will replace outdated and overworn equipment.

It makes no sense for our discussion to harp on horror stories of tubes being put down the wrong pipe or drug allergies being ignored. Lawyers don't get rich off anesthesia cases. Anesthesia is exceptionally safe and is getting safer all the time.

# Twenty-Four

# How Deep Will
# I Go Under?

*The eye sees a thing more clearly in
dreams than the imagination does
when awake.*

Leonardo da Vinci

» Medicine is not an exact science; it's an art which uses
science. The anesthesiologist may know how the body's
individual organs and systems may react to anesthetic
drugs and techniques, but very little is known about how
the actual *person* undergoing anesthesia reacts. For example, the anesthesiologist "knows" that the patient
under anesthesia does not *seem* to react to pain as he or
she would if awake. From the point of view of the surgical
personnel, the patient is "out" and feels no pain or any
other kind of sensation.

But beyond what the personal in the operating room
can see, medical science knows little about how deep the
patient actually goes while under general anesthesia. As a
result, sensation under anesthesia—even pain—remains
a controversial issue.

## Yardsticks

The anesthesiologist needs to steer a fine line between giving too much medication and not enough. Too much medication can impair the blood circulation, make it more difficult for the patient to begin breathing again, and make the recovery process slower. Too little, of course, opens up the possibility of both sensation and pain. So anesthesiologists have developed techniques to measure adequacy of anesthesia. With inhalation agents, for example, the minimal anesthetic concentration (or MAC) level is used. This is the concentration at which most people don't withdraw or pull away from an incision. The MAC level doesn't take into consideration the rare patient who needs much more. But again, this is a standard from the doctor's point of view. It doesn't really measure depth of anesthesia. It also doesn't take into consideration the use of muscle relaxants. A muscle relaxant will, after all, prevent the muscle from withdrawing upon incision and could mask the need for more anesthesia. Just because one drug induces a sleep-like state, while another relaxes the muscles, it doesn't mean the patient is properly anesthetized. If the two states are not in correct balance, the patient could still be too lightly anesthetized even though unable to move.

What complicates matters even more is the existence of what we call "implicit memory." This means that even though no direct, conscious recall of information occurs, there must be memory because of the evidence that *learning* has occurred. For example, in psychologist Henry Bennett's research, patients under anesthesia were told to touch their chins at the next postoperative interview. Later these patients touched their chins much more frequently than those from the control group. Yet the patients had no recollection of anything said to them in surgery.

There are other problems. Many of the signs of anesthesia getting lighter — tearing of the eyes, sweating, frowning, swallowing—are not easily seen when the patient is all covered up. Increased pulse and blood pressure, along with body movements (if the patient isn't paralyzed by muscle relaxants) are more noticeable signs.

> Depth of anesthesia is a mystery that perplexes the profession more than any other. Not only do we have no consistent yardstick, but we aren't really clear as to what we are trying to measure. One thing researchers are fairly sure of is that the depth of anesthesia will vary with different situations and different patients.

The isolated forearm technique, first developed by Professor Tunstall of Aberdeen University in Scotland, is an example of an attempt to scientifically measure depth of anesthesia. Here the flow of blood to one arm is cut off intermittently by a tourniquet, so the arm remains unaffected by the muscle relaxant. The patient might hold the doctor's or a nurse's hand until he or she goes to sleep. If the anesthesia gets too light, the patient will be able to use the "free" hand, either voluntarily or involuntarily, to signal that the anesthetic is wearing off. This is reassuring to both the patient and the anesthesiologist. Dr. Furlong has personally used this technique in cases where patients had complained of being "awake" during prior surgery.

Dr. Bennett has developed a machine that monitors facial muscle activity during surgery. The facial muscles seem to be less sensitive to the effects of muscle relaxants. Theoretically, then, they can indicate depth of anesthesia. The machine picks up barely perceptible contractions of the facial muscles. Increased activity in these muscles indicates lightening of anesthetic depth. Dr. Bennett even reported contraction of the smile muscles when he told a joke in the operating room.

Other techniques are undoubtedly just a few years away. The problem remains, however, that none of these techniques can actually get into the mind of the patient to truly measure the depth of anesthesia. Even though it's possible to measure the concentrations of anesthetic drugs in the blood, we can't yet determine the exact effect this has on the mind. We really don't yet have a foolproof method to measure depth of anesthesia.

As we shall see in later sections, patients who are seemingly lost to the world can still have a meaningful level of consciousness. They may feel pain at some level, and the pain may cause complications later. They may have memory of a sort. They may also have significant psychological reactions to what they hear while under anesthesia, and, as we shall see, these reactions can be either positive or negative.

# Twenty-Five

# Loose Lips Sink Ships

*Words, like eyeglasses, blur everything
that they do not make more clear.*

Joubert

» Unless a patient is undergoing eye surgery, the eyes will
be covered up and seeing will be impossible. But a
patient's ears are wide open through the entire surgical
process. The question is, then, can patients under general
anesthesia hear? The answer is, simply, yes.

Studies that monitor the brains of patients under
general anesthesia have found evidence of "hearing." The
anesthesia diminishes but does not abolish the electrical
activity in response to sound in the cerebral cortex —
*auditory-evoked potential*. The brain still responds to
sound.

But is the sound which reaches the brain meaningful?
Does it reach the brain in the form of words, or is it merely
a collection of electrical impulses? Patients all over the
world claim to hear and remember words, sentences, even
operating room dialogue. Since surgery can be a
psychologically difficult experience, the issue of hearing
during surgery is a sensitive one. It raises both problems
and possibilities.

A few real-life anecdotes will suffice to set the stage. A New York anesthesiologist, convinced that patients under general anesthesia were totally incapable of meaningful hearing, set out to prove his point by deliberately insulting his patient while she was "out." The woman was obese, and the comment related to her weight. Put briefly: she heard, she sued. Another New York anesthesiologist made the mistake of noting that her patient "was so fat, he had his own zip code." Fortunately the man had a sense of humor, and was satisfied with letting the doctor know he had heard the remark.

Incidents such as these may not be frequent, but they do occur. It's reasonable to infer that many more patients hear remarks made by surgical personnel in the operating room, but don't consciously remember the comments. The remarks, however, did reach the brain and were received—the damage of information received and retained subconsciously can be even worse than information the patients are able to remember.

> It's widely believed that patients can hear while under general anesthesia. What is worse, they can misinterpret stray remarks and operating-room small talk. Music or suggestion tapes can act as sound insulation. They can also pump in positive imagery.

The patient may wake up feeling anxious or upset, without knowing why. The remarks about obesity—or just plain nastiness—may seem unfortunate, but relatively harmless. But what about comments about medical matters such as the patient's prognosis, especially if it's not promising? A patient being wheeled into an operating room, not matter how well prepared, must be at least a little bit apprehensive. Why make matters worse?

For a person in this situation, even an innocent remark, possibly misunderstood, can cause an adverse psychological reaction. For example, one patient woke up from routine surgery absolutely petrified with anxiety. Fortunately the hospital had on staff a doctor with an interest in hypnosis. Under hypnosis, the patient said that she could hear the surgeon saying that he "couldn't get rid of the black spots." Naturally she thought that the surgeon had discovered some kind of incurable disease once he had opened her up. Upon questioning, the surgeon revealed that the unremovable black spots in question had not been on the patient at all, but on the surgeon's bathroom tiles.

The anecdote about the black spots may seem humorous, but it underscores a serious dilemma: when *you* go under anesthesia you (1) can't control what people say and (2) you may be oversensitive to what they do say. The fact that the information is likely to be "remembered" subconsciously can magnify the negative effect. Not everyone is as lucky as the woman with the "black spots." With the help of hypnosis, she was able to resolve what could have been a very serious problem. Hypnotic regression back to the time of surgery is not always possible. Nor is it always desirable, since it can itself be traumatic.

The premise of this book is getting a handle on "what goes into your body" and "what goes into your mind." The question of hearing under anesthesia is a prime component of the "what goes into your mind" part of our inquiry. As we shall soon discuss, you can affect what goes into your mind — through your wide-open ears — by using music and positive suggestions. Positive input may not filter out everything negative, but it will offer your brain a worthwhile alternative. Effective positive input can also consist of telling you to resist negative inputs. As we shall see, positive suggestions can themselves help you prepare for your surgery, and greatly enhance healing and recovery.

# Twenty-Six

# Do They Really Make the Pain Go Away?

*Pleasure is the absence of pain in the
body and of trouble in the soul.*

Epicurus

**»** Medical science can't state with certainty that "feeling"
does not occur during general anesthesia. The problem is
too complicated for an easy answer.

In regional or local anesthesia, for example, transmission of surgical stimuli to the brain is blocked. Thanks to
the anesthesia, it doesn't get past the pain gates. The
patient, who is conscious at the time, doesn't feel the pain,
since the stimulus never reaches the brain. Since the brain
is not involved, the pain simply does not exist. After local
anesthesia wears off, of course, there could be postsurgical
pain, but this is a different subject.

The story is different with general anesthesia. Consciousness *is* temporarily blocked, but the pain gates are
not. Pain can still get through to the brain, even though the
brain isn't aware and conscious of it. The manner in which
the higher centers of the brain process the stimuli caused
by the surgery is altered by the anesthesia. Memories of

the events of surgery are stored in some form but can't be recalled readily. Despite all this, the stimulus *does* get to the brain. Under normal consciousness this stimulus would be unbearably painful. Yet after general anesthesia, the patient will wake up and tell the doctor that he or she feels fine.

Certainly, from the doctor's point of view, the patient doesn't feel the pain of surgery. The patient doesn't move, cry out, or seem to react as if pain is being felt. The patient doesn't afterwards complain of having felt pain. The net result is that the general anesthesia process has taken the pain factor out of the operation. It has allowed the operation to proceed calmly.

If you interview the patient after surgery about sensation and pain, the patient will likely agree with the doctor: "I felt nothing." But this is the conscious mind speaking. From the point of view of the conscious mind, the pain never occurred, no matter what the surgeon may have done to the body.

> From the surgeon's point of view, you didn't "feel" pain during general anesthesia or you would have moved or cried out. Your own standard should be higher—you want your pain gates effectively blocked through modern, creative anesthetic techniques. Pain is too devastating to treat lightly.

But we humans are complex beings, with powerful and sensitive subconscious minds. While we don't react to the "pain" under general anesthesia as we would have, had we been conscious during surgery, the information does reach our brains in some form. While the consequences may not be serious or disturbing to us, at some point we have indeed registered the stimulus. We have "felt" something. Perhaps this is part of what doctors are talking about when they refer to the stress of surgery.

What we have felt may be so deeply buried that it has no effective meaning for us. For some, the consequences may be more far reaching. General anesthesia is a wonderful process that makes life-saving, life-enhancing surgery possible, but like all medical disciplines it's not an exact science. The question of whether pain is felt during general anesthesia can't be answered simply. If pain is felt, we must also examine the question of whether it's remembered.

# Twenty-Seven

# Thanks for the Memories

*Memory is the treasury and guardian of all knowledge.*

Cicero

>> Bob Hope might be grateful for all his memories, but most patients assume that they will remember nothing that happened to them while they were under general anesthesia. Of course we already know that the question of awareness under anesthesia is a complicated one. You might very well remember something. The question then remains: how does the memory affect you?

There are many explanations and theories of memory. They involve neurological and neurochemical processes and are constantly changing as new research is conducted.

*Short-term* and *long-term* memory are two distinct types. Short-term memory allows us to remember a telephone number long enough to dial it. Long term memory allows us to recall the number weeks later. Long-term memory can be recalled in great detail, especially if the event remembered is an exciting one—a wedding, the birth of a baby, graduation day. Other events may not be so clearly etched into memory.

Recall of stored memories can be enhanced by hypnosis. Hypnosis may help a witness to a crime remember details more vividly. Certain drugs, including those used in anesthesia, are known to either reduce or obliterate recall. But under hypnosis, some people can recall what happened, despite the drugs they were given during the surgery.

If a patient can describe actual words said during anesthesia, the anesthesia is generally considered inadequate. If light anesthesia is used along with muscle relaxants, the patient may seem to be fully anesthetized, but may actually be awake and unable to move. In the case of a cesarean operation, lighter levels of anesthesia are always preferred to protect the child being born. The mother is warned of the possibility of recall (though not of pain), both to reassure her and to prevent legal complaints. Patients undergoing heart bypass also need to be counseled that hearing may occur though pain is unlikely.

Even if you are "out cold" during surgery, it's likely that somewhere in your brain, somehow, you retain a memory of the event. By making sure your surgery takes place in a positive environment, you can safeguard yourself against mental impressions that can be damaging to you over the long term—often in subtle ways.

In England, a series of cases were reported where a number of patients in the same hospital were immobilized during surgery by muscle relaxants, but were actually wide awake—enough to feel and remember pain. These patients felt as if they had been chemically bound, gagged, and tortured. They formed a support group to try to deal with the severe posttraumatic stress disorder they were suffering. They described feelings of deep depression, insomnia, fear of death, and a very gloomy outlook on life. They were unable to function normally. Of course this kind of result among so many people is extremely rare.

Jeanette Tracy tells the harrowing story of her "routine" hernia operation in Texas; routine, that is, until the anesthetic gases ran out and left her paralyzed and unable to speak as her surgery was being performed. She remembers trying to cry, trying to scream, then feeling that a blowtorch was being applied to her stomach. "They couldn't hear me or sense what I was going through," she says. "I got through the experience by praying for my children."

Afterwards, Jeanette was so traumatized by her experience that she decided not to sue her doctors because a legal case would prevent her from telling her story so she could warn and protect others. The worst part was when the doctors told her it had all been her "imagination." But she then repeated operating room conversations—verbatim. She has since heard from hundreds of other people who have had similar experiences. Most have also been told they imagined the experience, but have been able to prove otherwise.

The usual case of recall is far less dramatic than Jeanette's, but there are still dangers. In cases of partial anesthesia, the patient may feel only a little pressure or remember a few words. Recall of painful sensations is rare. Nevertheless, any recall can be frightening if it takes the patient by surprise. As we have seen, anesthesiologists still don't have an absolutely reliable way to measure depth of anesthesia. If they did, most cases such as Jeanette's could be avoided.

The most common example of patient awareness is in the case of trauma—an accident or sudden injury. When a patient is suffering from severe blood loss, the main emphasis is on keeping the patient alive. Initial anesthesia is usually light. Perhaps muscle relaxants alone will be used, as the trauma victim may have dangerously low blood pressure. As the patient begins to come to, however, he or she may begin to feel pain. Patients react differently to this. Some are grateful to the rescuers. Some see them as the cause of their pain.

In many cases the delay in giving adequate anesthesia is a judgment call by an inexperienced resident. In any case of light anesthesia, the doctor should say something to the patient to try to relieve the patient's terror. The patient may already be terrified of dying. He or she can do without the added fear of being undermedicated.

Dr. David Cheek, an obstetrician and gynecologist, used hypnosis to prepare his patients for surgery and childbirth. He also treated patients who were suffering from neurotic complexes after surgery. Some had recurring nightmares; others had unexpected pain or an irrational fear of cancer that caused weight loss. Some had poor wound healing. Dr. Cheek helped these patients to reach a deep state of hypnosis and regress to the time of surgery. To his amazement, they started telling him what had been said in the operating room, often in great detail. For many, the process helped uncover and resolve the cause of the distress. An example: a doctor who used the word "cancer" even though the condition later turned out to be benign. Unfortunately, few patients get a chance to be hypnotized to find out that their fears were based on stray words or misunderstandings. Dr. Cheek understood that the best treatment is always prevention. He wanted operating rooms to post signs reading "THE PATIENT CAN HEAR YOU." But few doctors heeded his advice.

Psychiatrist Bernard Levinson heard about Cheek's work. The two corresponded and theorized that events of a frightening nature would be more likely to be imprinted in the mind than neutral events. Levinson selected ten hypnotizable subjects who were to have dental surgery. During the surgery, at a signal, the anesthesiologist said, "Stop the surgery. The patient is blue." After giving the patient more oxygen, the anesthesiologist would say, "You may continue. Everything is OK now." This was said at the deepest levels of ether anesthesia that could be gone to safely.

None of the patients had any recall of the utterances after the surgery. But one month later, under hypnosis, four of the ten patients told exactly what had been said, four others could say that something had gone wrong, and two could not enter the state necessary to get the information.

The experiences of Cheek and Levinson show that recording of events, feelings, sensations, and words under anesthesia is a real possibility. It's not easy to predict whether the imprinting will be damaging. It's best to be on the safe side by asking your surgeon to avoid negative comments in the operating room and by using positive inputs such as music and suggestion cassettes. Whether or not you are allowed to use cassettes while under anesthesia, you should tell yourself that you will respond only to positive words spoken directly to you.

# Twenty-Eight

# The Power of Suggestions During Surgery

*The power of Thought, the magic of the Mind!*

**Byron**

**»** We've established that hearing and sensation are possible during general anesthesia. Variations of memory have also been reported. Clearly the mind, at least on a subconscious level, is hard at work during surgery, and it's a powerful mind.

Years ago subliminal advertising messages were successfully used in movie theaters. A message such as "Buy Popcorn" would be flashed on the screen too briefly for the conscious mind to register it. The conscious mind remembered nothing of the message, yet snack bar sales increased just the same. The technique proved to be so compelling that it was quickly banned from television and cinema.

Over the decades, researchers in many disciplines have continued to investigate legitimate uses of the subconscious. Suggestions have been used to alter unhealthy eating habits, to relax patients so as to lower their blood pressure, to reduce pain, and to help people quit smoking. To say the mind has an effect on the body is already outdated — the mind and body are truly one. So what goes into our brains also goes into our bodies, at least in some form. In scientific terms, the mind-body connection is a difficult thing to prove, but any doctor will tell you that patients who want to survive serious illnesses, people who have a real will to live, will stand a better chance of surviving than people who allow themselves to be consumed by their fears and negative thoughts.

All through this book we've been stressing the importance of attitude and positive thought as an antidote to fear, worry and pain. Let's leave general theory behind for a moment. It helps a lot to understand how and why something works. But you also need to know what to do too. So what can you do to fill up your brain with helpful images while you're under? The answer is, play audio suggestion tapes. You can buy them ready-made. Or, as we'll see in the next chapter, you can make your own.

Anesthesiologists and researchers who are interested in improving patient response to surgery have had growing success in using subliminal suggestions on patients under general anesthesia. The goals have been generally to reduce anxiety, to enhance healing, to help manage pain, and to reduce the complications of anesthesia and surgery.

Early studies by Dr. Pearson and Dr. Wolff were quite encouraging. In Dr. Pearson's study, patients who received positive suggestions went home from the hospital earlier than usual. In Dr. Wolff's study patients had fewer complaints of pain. Evans and Richardson, in a controlled study, also reported patients going home earlier. Furlong and McClintock reported reduced need for pain medication by their suggestion group. Other studies have yielded a variety of positive results—from reduced anxiety to a lower level of postsurgical sore throat.

> Patients who listen to audiotapes of therapeutic suggestions while they're under general anesthesia often show encouraging results: less pain, shorter hospital stays, and a more positive outlook. Interest in suggestion tapes is growing in many circles as doctors come to realize the importance of mental and emotional factors in healing.

Other studies didn't show improvement. There are many possible explanations for this. Patients are not equally capable of responding to suggestions. Some patients may be responding in ways that are not being measured or that have not been anticipated. Some patients in the control group (the ones who don't receive any suggestions) may have such a positive outlook all on their own—without any suggestions—that they skew the results of the experiment. Some patients may have been accidentally exposed to negative comments even though they are in a controlled study. Many of the experiment groups may still be too small to give meaningful results. So it's not easy to draw final conclusions.

Until many more controlled experiments are conducted, researchers will not say for certain that suggestions really work. But in the real world, both the doctors who prescribe them and the patients who listen to them have reason to be excited about suggestions. People were getting tremendous benefits from aspirin and penicillin long before controlled experiments were done. Anecdotal evidence from all over the world is very encouraging about using positive suggestions.

As we shall see, there are two kinds of tapes. The one we've been talking about takes you through the actual surgery. But there's another to help you through the conscious process of preparing yourself for surgery.

## Suggestions Before Surgery

The presurgical tape covers getting yourself ready. It helps you resolve possible fears and uncertainties. The presurgical tape also guides your imagery toward a positive outcome — straight through the operating room, into the recovery room, back to the hospital room, then back home.

The presurgical tape covers more ground and is longer than the surgical tape. Here's an example of a pre-surgical tape text that's effective:

*Find a comfortable position.*

*Take a few deep breaths in through your nose and, more slowly, out through your mouth. Roll your eyes up as far as they will go.*

*As your eyelids become heavy, just take a deep breath, and as you breathe out slowly close your eyes and let them relax.*

*There's nothing special you have to do now. Enjoy the music for a while. Enjoy the warm feeling of having nothing to do, just taking time for you alone.*

*Perhaps you would like to imagine going to an especially comfortable place, somewhere you are warm, comfortable, and relaxed, like a quiet beach. First let's start on a path down from a hilltop to find out where your mind wants to go. This will be your favorite place. You'll do your mental preparation for surgery here.*

*OK now—you're on the hilltop. It's a nice day. The sun is shining, and there's a pleasantly cool breeze blowing, bringing the scents of flowers. Walk down the winding pathway, leading through trees. See the dappled light. Feel the crunch of bracken and pine cones. Smell the pines and other scents.*

*Your mind wants to choose where you will go—perhaps to a beach or a lovely garden. As you move further down the path, you come to some stairs. Slowly walk down, noticing each step as you go deeper down. You see a tall hedge of trees and beyond the trees is your special place. How do you get through the hedge? Is there a gate or an archway?*

*Enter your special place. Look around. What is it like? Here we are going to work. Take a little time to look around and find a comfortable place to rest.*

*Are there any birds singing? Are there any flowers? What colors are they? What scents do they have?*

*Doing mental preparation for surgery is easy and helps you heal faster and more comfortably. There is no right way to do it. Just follow these instructions in your own way. This is your unique experience.*

*You are finding out as much as you need to know about surgery and anesthesia and the ways the doctors and nurses can keep you comfortable after the operation.*

*During anesthesia you are safe and protected. Everything goes well. You are in skilled caring hands. During surgery your mind can go to any place, like the place you are now. Your protective healing mind is already programmed to automat-*

*ically take over, so you don't have to worry about not being in control. You are not concerned with conversations in the operating room. You only respond subconsciously to healing words spoken directly to you. When your operation is over, you open your eyes and breathe with ease when it's time to do so. You feel calm and relaxed because you know the healing part of your mind is already directing your recovery from surgery and getting you ready to leave the hospital healthy and happy, as soon as possible.*

*Think for a moment about your favorite food. Maybe it's the food your mother made when you stayed home from school with a cold. After your surgery, thinking of this encourages your peristalsis (the waves your stomach and bowels make) to go the right way, so anything in the stomach goes down, not up.*

*If in the past you vomited after anesthesia, just acknowledge what a strongly protective reaction your body had. Now you know that you don't need to vomit at all. All the substances your doctors and nurses give you are removed either by your lungs, your liver, or your kidneys, so your stomach can have a rest.*

*Much of the discomfort after surgery is due to swelling and muscle spasm. We don't often exercise this power, but we all have the ability to relax muscles and reduce swelling. Think of the muscles relaxing, and they will relax more and more with practice. Also practice using your arms to lift yourself if you are having an incision in the tummy area. To protect your stomach, you can hug a pillow if you need to cough.*

*You can even redirect the flow of blood away from the site of your operation by imagining a cool feeling in this area to reduce sensation, bleeding, and swelling. Later your blood will flow back just enough to bring healing oxygen and nourishing proteins to the area of surgery. Your body knows how to do this and responds to your mental images.*

*All these activities are energized by a beautiful healing light. Feel the warm light and notice the colors.*

*Now, just touch your left little finger to your left palm. You can do this during the day, to quickly bring back this feeling of relaxation and remind yourself of the images you are creating.*

*Also during the day, you can repeat an affirmation to yourself such as "I am safe, I heal wonderfully."*

*In the recovery room you are not disturbed by the activity around you. You are perfectly comfortable with any special equipment in use for your support. You wave your arm for attention if needed.*

*You feel calm and relaxed. Relaxing the muscles around the area of surgery helps you feel comfortable and helps any medicine you may need work better.*

*Back in your room you continue to feel relaxed. You can decide if you want to take the medicine your doctors have ordered to help you be more comfortable. Whatever you decide is safe and OK.*

*Now is a good time to see yourself doing the things you want to do when you return home and are completely healed. Memories of your hospitalization fade more and more as time goes by. It's so good to make plans for the future.*

*Open your mind to accept the highest powers of your mind to help you heal. They know just what to do.*

*If you wish to go to sleep after the tape, continue to close your eyes and sleep well. End the tape here.*

*If you want to wake up, I'll count you out slowly.*

*5—Still warm and relaxed.*

*4—Getting ready to have a good day.*

*3—Fingers and toes feel tingly, getting ready for action.*

*2—Coming up slowly, breathing nice and evenly now.*

*1—Wide awake feeling fine, relaxed, and more and more healthy each day.*

*Wake up now. May all be well with you.*

## Suggestions During Surgery

A tape text for use during surgery will involve an auto-reverse continuous-play personal stereo machine so the suggestions can recycle and repeat. This text is much simpler than the presurgical text. Essentially, it contains reassuring positive statements about safety, not paying attention to extraneous comments, waking up feeling calm and relaxed, having good postoperative results, and general suggestions for health and happiness. There is no set text. Because you'll be asleep when the tape will be played, be sure to have the anesthesiologist set the tape volume to a comfortably low level.

As we shall see in the next chapter, the most powerful tape text may be one you create yourself.

# Twenty-Nine

# Writing Your Own Suggestions

*Words are but pictures of our thoughts.*

**Dryden**

≫ One of Dr. Furlong's patients was extremely distressed about having her breast removed for cancer. She wrote her own suggestions, which Dr. Furlong read to her while she was under general anesthesia. The following is her script:

*You will be OK mentally and physically after the operation.*

*You will be up and about and out of bed very soon. You will still be a whole person, as good as new and just as feminine as ever.*

*It will not be horrible to look at yourself. It will be all right. You will be all right because you are very strong. You will make it through the ordeal and come out a winner.*

*It will be hard at first, but you will pull up your inner resources and you will make it. The sun will shine again, and you will be able to enjoy life.*

*The inner emotional pain will chill with time, and you will feel even better than before because you will take the time to reach within.*

*When you awake, you will not feel as depressed as you think you might. You will be able to handle this because you are strong—stronger than you know. You will get through this and on with your life and within time your life will be happy.*

*You will see the light at the end of the tunnel, and you will make it there—the inner child and you.*

> Writing your own suggestions—even using your own voice on the suggestion tape—is simply a fabulous idea. You get a chance to reinforce your own positive thoughts when you listen to the tape. But even better, the *process* of creating suggestions to be played back or read to you under general anesthesia maximizes your personal involvement in the surgical process.

Using a pre-recorded suggestion tape is valuable, but you should consider writing your own suggestions as well. The value of writing your own suggestions is that they address your own particular concerns. A good way to start is by writing down your concerns in a notebook. The process of writing is important; you might come up with some things you hadn't thought about before.

The purpose of the suggestions is to give affirmations and encouragement instead of repeating and reinforcing the worries. It's important to look at the worries and do everything practical to answer them. At the same time, you can make positive affirmations. Following is an example of the tape Dr. Furlong uses for her patients. It's a good starting point for your own efforts to customize the suggestions you will hear.

*Listen to my voice. Listen only to my voice and the music, as you feel safe and secure.*

*Though you are deeply asleep, you hear and respond to my voice.*

*Don't be concerned with conversations in the operating room. Listen only to those words spoken directly to you. You are safe, protected and in life-sustaining hands. Your bodily functions are stable. Your physical condition is improving. All is well. Listen only to words spoken directly to you. You are safe and secure.*

*When the operation is over, you will wake up feeling calm and relaxed. You will open your eyes and take a deep breath. You will feel as if you are resting in your own bed. You will be at ease with the activity around you. Your throat will be clear, and you will breathe easily.*

*You will be pleasantly hungry and thirsty. You will empty your bladder and bowels easily and in good time. There will be a gentle, warm sensation in the area of your operation, and you will be able to move comfortably.*

*Any memory of discomfort is fading and will soon be gone. Positive thoughts will help you to heal quickly, go home early, and stay healthy. From this day forward, your thoughts will be: I am healing completely. I take care of myself by getting enough rest, eating nourishing food, and enjoying life. I am healthy and happy. All is well.*

Because the subconscious can take things literally, give simple directions. Use affirmative phrases such as You will feel comfortable, instead of negative instructions like You will feel no pain. The process of creating the script is itself valuable. As soon as you write the statement, you are sending the right message to your mind, even if you never get to play the suggestions during the operation. But for optimal results, work hard on your suggestions. Try to make them cover your major concerns and arrange to listen to them while under anesthesia.

# Thirty

# Healing

*Healing is a matter of time, but it is sometimes also a matter of opportunity.*

Hippocrates

» The healing process is a holistic one. It involves both mind and body. It begins, not in the recovery room, but before you ever enter the hospital. The healing process can also continue for a very long time after you leave the hospital. You may be facing the prospect of radiation therapy or up to a year of chemotherapy. If you're recovering from orthopedic surgery you may need a long course of physical therapy. You'll definitely need to keep your spirits up while you go through this difficult time in your life. A positive experience, both in surgery and immediately after, will be a good base for your entire healing process.

You enter the hospital not to become ill, but to become well. Becoming well is your job, and we've discussed many things you can do to get the job done. First and foremost, you will take control of what goes into your body and what goes into your mind. Your goal is to control and manage pain. We've already discussed some techniques.

Pain is not a phenomenon with a beginning and an end. Pain has lasting effects. It can retard and reverse healing. It can rob you of your sleep and sap the strength your body needs to recuperate from the trauma of surgery. It can prevent you from breathing properly and from eating properly. If pain prevents you from walking, problems such as blood clots can result.

But the worst aspect of pain is the stress to your whole system, to the mind-body continuum. Pain brings in its wake fear, stress, a thousand negative emotions. Freedom from pain is the linchpin to healing.

Here is where your outlook comes in. It's very important for you to have clear plans for the future. Like holding out the carrot in front of the donkey, you'll create an incentive to act as a carrot for your subconscious mind. This comes in the form of a clear mental picture of the things you will be doing after you have healed. It begins with a visualization of yourself in the recovery room, reacting well to the surgery, and proceeds to you leaving the hospital, going home, and resuming the activities you enjoy doing. A good pre-op relaxation tape will guide you through this process.

Keeping a journal helps you work on your outlook effectively. A refinement on the journal is to make a life-plan chart (which is useful in all aspects of life, not just surgery) to define where you are and where you are going. Write these headings on the tops of four separate journal pages: *Health, Love and Relationships, Material Concerns*, and *Creative Self-Expression*. On the *Health* page you'll put down your thoughts and desires about your body (including your weight), the clothing size you'd like to be, and any other concerns. Under *Love and Relationships* you'll analyze where you want your relationships to go. This includes romantic love, children, and friends. If you're looking for an ideal mate, you'll put down all the details here. *Material Concerns* covers how much money you want to make, save, or invest. You should be ambitious here; try to expand your financial expectations. Finally, *Creative Self-Expression* deals with your own goals for your work, your interests, and the enrichment of your life. The process of creating the life-plan chart is not only extremely valuable, it's uplifting and positive. Many people who have used it say that it works and helps make dreams come true.

Mind and body are not only connected, they are in fact one. They combine to form you. We've seen that the brain *creates* pain rather than merely registering it. We've also seen how the brain blocks pain. In the same way, if your brain is working for you and not against you, every other physical process involving healing will be enhanced. It pays, then, to take steps to remain emotionally well throughout the surgery and its aftermath. Full access to information, support from family and friends, the use of suggestion tapes, music, the comforts of home – all these things can combine to enhance your wellness. Without these extras, you're just a case number.

It's not that medical personnel are uncaring, but they are busy. Their work demands that when they finish with you, they move on to someone else. Most medical people want to pay more attention to their patients, but the structure under which they work doesn't allow it. Nearly all financial resources in medicine come from insurance. The lion's share of the money tends to support complicated technical procedures rather than time-consuming person-to-person contact. Until the system itself changes to allow medical people more time to interact with patients, only you and the people you love can ensure that you obtain the optimum resources for healing.

Even if those resources are optimum and your healing process goes splendidly, you still must live with your body's physical limitations. When can you resume your normal activities? An exercise routine? The answer to these questions vary with the surgery. It's important – with your doctor's help — to find the right period of convalescence for you. Pampering yourself with bed rest can be carried too far. On the other hand, especially with minor surgery, you do run the risk of getting back into the swing of things too soon if you're active in athletics.

> Healing requires a good mix of positive mind-set, on the one hand, and outright pampering, on the other. While your body will need to rest after surgery, your brain and your emotions should be moving forward in a positive direction.

Surgery is a traumatic shock to the system, even if the incision is small and the operation brief. The anesthesia and other medications you have been given will take time to work their way through your system. Your metabolism will take a few days to get back to normal. Your body will not be able to deliver nutrients to the muscles efficiently for a while. The hormonal changes surgery brings on can take a good few weeks to normalize. The surgical wound, even if small, can also take a few weeks to heal properly through the action of collagen — the body's glue — and scar tissue.

Professional athletes have been known to exercise the same day after undergoing arthroscopic surgery — but remember, they are paid enormous sums of money to perform at that level. If you are a serious amateur athlete, you must be prepared to slow down a bit to really heal. Even though you are away from your exercise routines, you can visualize doing the exercises. When the proper time comes, you can resume your athletics and perhaps do better than ever. No matter how well you are doing emotionally, it's important to respect your body's time table.

Your task in healing is to know your body, know your mind, know *yourself* — and take care of yourself accordingly.

Of course the healing doesn't always go as we plan — and it can be frustrating. For example, one of Dr. Furlong's patients was scheduled to have his stomach removed. He was enthusiastic about being part of a study where he would listen to a cassette tape of suggestions during surgery. The anesthesia went well, but the operation didn't. The surgeon found that the patient's cancer had spread and that means to treat the cancer, other than surgery, were now preferred. The patient was understandably depressed, but over a longer term he did wonderfully. He had laser surgery and chemotherapy and tolerated both very well. He went back to work and even went on a second honeymoon. His is the perfect story of an involved patient. He believed in the mind-body connection, read inspirational books, welcomed the tapes, and did everything that he could to heal himself through very difficult circumstances, including postsurgical depression.

# Transcending the Emotional Limits

*Growth is the only evidence of life.*
John Henry Newman

» Pain, illness, healing, and recovery are extreme events in this drama we call human life. As with any extreme, they pose dangers, but they also give us the seeds of opportunity to change and to grow. When we go through a healing process, the emotional factor is as important as the physical. Physically, we can heal to the extent that we make ourselves whole again—we make our bodies back into what they were. Emotionally, however, we can go much farther—we can grow way beyond what we were when we started the process.

Personal emotional growth simply has no limits. Like a tough physical workout, an emotional challenge can leave us stronger than before. We can find surprising strength and resilience in adversity. Beating pain — and we have seen exactly how we can do this — can be a particularly formative experience.

Take the example of a woman plagued by chronic pain. Medications just don't seem to work. She begins to keep a regular journal, writing every night for an hour or so. As time goes on, she gets more emotionally involved with the journal, looking forward during the day for the moment she can put all her cares aside and get back to her writing, to her self-exploration.

It doesn't hit her all at once. But over the months she comes to realize that when she is working on her journal, when she is emotionally charged up, she doesn't feel the pain. In fact, the beneficial effect lasts long after she stops writing. A positive has canceled out a negative. Mind and body have worked together to evolve a way out of a physical threat to well-being.

Norman Cousins' battle against serious illness is well known. His remedy was laughter. He found that if he kept laughing, he just didn't have the time to feel ill. Death finally caught up with him — at age 75 — but his self-evolved techniques undoubtedly added years to his life. Cousins called the immune system a "mirror to life" that reflects all its joys and anguish. Cousins wasn't a scientist, of course, and scientists demand more rigorous proofs than he did. Yet he must have known his body, just as we ought to know ours.

Scientists are moving on some of the same tracks as Cousins, investigating the mind-body link and how it relates to healing and wellness. A study at Stanford University Medical School during the 1980s found that women with advanced breast cancer who received group psychotherapy as well as medical treatment lived significantly longer than a similar group who received no psychotherapy.

Dr. Bernie Siegel is perhaps the most widely followed proponent of the mind-body link. His work stresses the idea that we should strive to live to our fullest potential. It's important to think for ourselves. It's important to reach for what is fulfilling for us, not what our religion, our society, or our parents want for us. Dr. Siegel talks of people diagnosed with serious diseases who change their life styles because they are sure they're going to die. Yet because of the change, they find they are just beginning to live. And often they do live far beyond the few years their doctors have given them.

> Even when your life is threatened by disease or difficult medical procedures, you have a window of opportunity for personal growth and inner healing. On the other hand, if you give in to worry and fear, your body gets the message. It's definitely a chemical message: one that can depress the immune system, raise your cholesterol, and do other sorts of damage to you. Emotions are chemical reactions.

Faced with illness — if we deny our needs, if we don't live genuinely — the body mechanism that deals with physical change gets the negative message. Things go from bad to worse. We become oriented toward disease and death.

Dr. Siegel would be first to admit that he is not infallible and that much of his work is unproven. But the application for the surgical patient is clear: learn to get in touch with yourself, pinpoint your emotional needs and difficulties, treat yourself exceptionally well.

Rather than see your hospital stay as a challenge, try to view it as an opportunity. Maybe you have been running from pain all your life — this is the time to stand and fight. Maybe you've never quite understood who you are and what you want out of life — this is the time to do a little thinking. Maybe there is something particular you really want to resolve inside yourself, but you just haven't had the time. You do now—while you're healing. Your routine has changed, your surroundings have changed, your thoughts are going in new directions—it's time to make some progress in your life—it's time to grow just a little bit.

# Thirty-Two

# Epilogue—What You Put in Your Body

*It is best to rise from life as from a banquet, neither thirsty nor drunken.*
Aristotle

➤ Aristotle's advice about life also applies to surgery. Ultimately, *you* are responsible for what medications they put into your body—and how much. Yes, they (the doctors) do know more about medications than you do. But *you* know more about your body and the pain it feels than they do. *You* are the one who will suffer if the mix of medications is not adequate. They will already be treating the next patient.

You have three main stumbling blocks to ensuring adequate pain medication. Lack of communication is the first, but that's something you have some control over. Physician and nurse prejudice against the use of narcotics is second. More subtle, perhaps more dangerous, is the widespread belief among physicians that the patient can "tough it out," that some pain can even be formative—like the cold baths they prescribe for boys at elite English boarding schools.

The nineteenth century is long over. In fact, the twentieth century is nearly over. There is no place in modern medicine for such backward thinking. Yet you might find it. You've got to guard against it, communicate your needs, insist on your rights. Surgery is tough enough without having to endure unnecessary pain. No one has the right to let you suffer based on thinking that has long since been discredited.

> Mental and emotional techniques are essential for controlling postsurgical pain, but only one out of every ten patients can completely control severe pain by mind alone. Most people need some form of medication. Doing without drugs is a worthwhile goal. But if you need help from a drug, it doesn't make you any worse a person.

Drug abuse is a real problem in society today. But there is another side of the coin. *Hysteria* is not too light a word to use about the attitude some people have to drugs. The airwaves, milk cartons, grocery bags, the backs of telephone books all resound with the slogan "Just Say No to Drugs." It has never been proven that truly addictive personalities are affected by these slogans. Everyone else does pay attention, however, and unnecessary surgical pain is often the result.

A problem, yes, but there are two truths that must guide you. First, you will need some narcotics. Second, narcotic addiction among otherwise normal surgical patients is almost unknown. Once you work out your own possible antipathy towards narcotics, you can begin to insist on your rights. If the doctor begins to give you a story that seems to reflect a hardened anti-narcotic line, you must be prepared to counter it from a position of knowledge. Don't be afraid to stress to the doctor that "this is my pain, not yours."

Mental and emotional techniques are very important in controlling and eliminating pain. They undoubtedly decrease the need for drugs. But they are usually used in conjunction with drugs, not instead of drugs. They help the narcotics to work and activate your other healing mechanisms at the same time. But only ten to thirty percent of postsurgical patients (depending on the nature of the surgery) can do without drugs entirely.

# Thirty-Three

# Epilogue—What You Put in Your Mind

*There is nothing either good or bad, but thinking makes it so.*

William Shakespeare

» Hamlet, Shakespeare's greatest creation, has given us these remarkable words. Hamlet insists that *he* makes his world; as *he* views it, so it is. Attitude is everything. In the same way, preparing to undergo surgery, *we* make *our* world. It can be a world of calm control, of intelligent choice, of getting in touch with our emotions and our bodies. It can also be a world of fear, worry, pain, and anxiety. The choice is ours.

The subconscious mind is powerful, and it has a powerful effect on our perception of pain. Positive and negative inputs into the conscious mind also have their effect on the subconscious. The conscious mind is also mighty handy for processing information and making decisions. As we have seen, if you want quality pain management, you have to absorb a good deal of information and make quite a few crucial decisions. In addition, you've got to send what is in your mind to other minds. It's called communication.

Screening out negative thoughts and images is good. Putting in positive thoughts and images is better. We've discussed many ways to stay positive, like keeping a calm environment, doing self-developmental work before and after surgery, cementing support networks, gaining confidence by becoming a knowledgeable medical consumer. But the most sensitive moments of all come to us when we are actually under general anesthesia. We've been wheeled into an unfamiliar room filled with machinery, sedated, put on artificial respiration, forced into a sleep-like state and then, as if this weren't bad enough, someone starts cutting into us with a scalpel! It's at this critical moment that an inpouring of nourishing thoughts and images can be so helpful.

> Keep your thoughts — and the outside stimuli that affect your thoughts — going in the right direction, and you will have a solid mental and emotional base for getting through surgery, with the finest possible results.

By using a suggestion tape during surgery, you are ensuring that your brain is properly fed, adequately fortified for the shock your system is undergoing. You can't negate that shock by rational thinking alone. You — mind and body — have to become fully involved. You must bring emotions and passions into the equation. It's all a struggle to maintain your vital life force, to safeguard your health against any threat. It's a matter of active will — all within the realm of possibility.

There is nothing magic or unscientific about the will to live. It's a will *to live well*, to do something more than merely survive. Bare survival means accepting pain and grief. We humans demand more than that. We demand health, the true enjoyment of life. And it comes from within us.

We all have the will to get the most out of life somewhere inside us. Some of us have to dig a little deeper than others to find it. But find it we must. It's truly the only lasting solution to the problems of illness, fear, and pain.

As the surgical patient, *you* are the final controller of your own experience. Because information in the field of anesthesia and surgery is constantly changing, it's very important to listen carefully to all the information your doctors give you. That way, you and your doctors can make the best decisions together — as partners in your surgical care.

But some things don't change with technology: you, your healing abilities, the mind's effect on the body. The more you use the inner healing skills you already have, the better you will respond to your medical treatment.

# Suggested Readings

Achterberg, Jeanne. *Imagery in Healing*. Boston: Shambhala, 1985.

Ader, R.; Felten, D.L.; Cohen, N. *Psychoneuroimmunology* (2nd ed.). New York: Academic Press, 1991.

Agency for Health Care Policy and Research, U.S. Department of Health and Human Services. *Pain Control After Surgery: A Patient's Guide*, Publication No. AHCPR91-0021, Feb. 1992.

Alvarez, Elizabeth, and Fuchs, Sharon. "Bouncing Back From Surgery." *Health*, March 1987 v19 p49(4).

American Society of Anesthesiologists. *When Your Child Needs Surgery*. Park Ridge, IL: ASA.

Antonovsky, Aaron. *Health, Stress, and Coping*. San Francisco: Jossey-Bass, 1979.

Barsky, Arthur J. *Worried Sick: Our Troubled Quest for Wellness*. New York: Little, Brown, 1988.

Bennett, Hal, and Samuels, Mike. *The Well Body Book*. New York: Random House, 1973.

Benson, Herbert. *The Mind/Body Effect*. New York: Simon & Schuster, 1979

Benson, Herbert. *The Relaxation Response*. New York: William Morrow, 1975.

Bonke, Benno; Fitch, William; and Millar, Keith. *Memory and Awareness in Anaesthesia*. Rockland, MA: Swets & Zeitlinger, 1990.

Borysenko, Joan. *Minding the Body, Mending the Mind*. New York, Bantam Books, 1988.

Boyd, Hamish. *Introduction to Homeopathic Medicine*. New Canaan, CT: Keats Publishing, 1981.

Bresler, David E., and Turbo, Richard. *Free Yourself From Pain*. New York: Simon & Schuster, 1979.

Bronson, Gail. "A Consumer's Guide to Making Your Surgery as Painless as Possible." *American Health: Fitness of Body and Mind*, April 1991 v10 n3 p33(7)

Campbell, Don (ed.). *Music Physician: For Times to Come*. Wheaton, IL: Quest Books, 1991.

Cohen, Sheldon, and Syme, S. Leonard (eds.). *Social Support and Health*. New York: Academic Press, 1985.

Corey, David, with Soloman, Stan. *Pain: Free Yourself for Life*. New York: NAL-Dutton, 1989.

Cousins, Norman. *Anatomy of an Illness*. New York: W.W. Norton, 1979.

Cousins, Norman. *The Healing Heart*. New York: Avon Books, 1984.

Cousins, Norman. *Head First: The Biology of Hope and the Healing Power of the Human Spirit*. New York: Viking Penguin, 1990.

Dachman, Ken, and Lyons, John. *You Can Relieve Pain*. New York: Harper Perennial, 1990.

Dienstfrey, Harris. *Where the Mind Meets the Body*. New York: Harper-Collins, 1991.

Dossey, Larry. *Space, Time & Medicine*. Boston: New Science Library, 1982.

Dubos, René. *Mirage of Health*. New York: Doubleday, 1959.

Egbert, L.D.; Battit, G.E.; Turndorf H; et al. "The Value of the Preoperative Visit by an Anesthetist." *Journal of the American Medical Association* 185:553, 1963.

Epstein, Gerald N. *Healing Visualization: Creating Health Through Imagery*. New York: Bantam, 1989.

Feltman, John (ed.). *Hands-On Healing: Massage Remedies for Hundreds of Health Problems*. Emmaus, PA: Rodale Press, 1989.

Fields, H.L. *Pain*, 1987.

Frank, Jerome. *Persuasion and Healing*. Baltimore: Johns Hopkins Press, 1973.

Gallo, Nick. "Kinder, Gentler Surgery: Less Pain, Faster Recovery, Lower Cost." *Better Homes and Gardens*, Sept 1992 v70 n9 p64(3).

Gentry, Doyle W. (ed.). *Handbook of Behavioral Medicine*. New York: The Guilford Press, 1984.

Goleman, Daniel. *The Meditative Mind: The Varieties of Meditative Experience*. Los Angeles, J.P. Tarcher, 1990.

Goleman, Daniel, and Gurin, Joel (eds.). *Mind Body Medicine: How to Use Your Mind for Better Health*. Yonkers, NY: Consumer Reports Books, 1993.

Gordon, James S. *Stress Management*. New York: Chelsea House, 1990.

Gordon, James S; Jaffee, Dennis; Bresler, David (eds.). *Mind, Body and Health: Toward an Integral Medicine*. New York: Human Sciences Press, 1984.

Guerra, Frank, and Aldrete, J. Antonio (eds.). *Emotional and Psychological Responses to Anesthesia and Surgery*. New York: Grune & Stratton, 1980.

Hausman, Patricia and Hurley, Judith Benn. *The Healing Foods: The Ultimate Authority on the Curative Power of Nutrition*. Emmaus, PA: Rodale Press, 1989.

Hay, Louise. *You Can Heal Your Life*. Santa Monica, CA: Hay House, 1987.

Hilgard, E.R.; Hilgard, J.R. *Hypnosis in the Relief of Pain*. Los Altos, CA: William Kaufman, 1975.

Hendler, N., and Fenton, J.A. *Coping With Chronic Pain*. New York: Clarkson N. Potter, 1979.

House, J.S.; Landis, K.R.; and Umberson, D. "Social Relationships and Health," *Science*, 241(1988):540-545.

Jaffe, Dennis T. *Healing From Within: Psychological Techniques to Help the Mind Heal the Body*. New York: Simon & Schuster, 1986.

Janis, I.L. *Psychological Stress, Psychoanalytic and Behavioral Studies of Surgical Patients*. New York: John Wiley & Sons, 1958.

Jones, J.G. (ed.). "Depth of Anesthesia." *Ballière's Clinical Anaesthesiology: International Practice and Research*, vol 3, no 3, December 1989.

Kabat-Zinn, Jon. *Full Catastrophe Living: Using the Wisdom of Your Body and Mind to Face Stress, Pain and Illness*. New York: Delacorte, 1991.

Kerr, F.W.L. *The Pain Book*, 1981.

Klein, Allen. *The Healing Power of Humor*. New York: Tarcher/Perigee, 1989.

Kowalchik, Claire and Hylton, William (eds.). *Rodale's Illustrated Encyclopedia of Herbs*. Emmaus, PA: Rodale Press, 1987.

Lipton and Sampson. *Conquering Pain*, 1984.

Locke, Steven E., and Colligan, Douglas. *The Healer Within: The New Medicine of Mind and Body*. New York: NAL-Dutton, 1987.

Matarazzo, Joseph D.; Weiss, Sharlene M.; Herd, J. Alan; Miller, Neal E.; and Weiss, Stephen M. (eds.). *Behavioral Health*. New York: John Wiley, 1984.

McCarthy, Laura Flynn. "Far from the Medical Mainstream." *Cosmopolitan*, Nov 1992 v213 n5 p262(5).

McKeown, Thomas. *The Role of Medicine: Dream, Mirage or Nemesis?* Princeton, NJ: Princeton University Press, 1979.

McLoed, Beverly. "Rx for Health: A Dose of Self-Confidence; The Mind Can Help the Body Mend When You Learn to Cope With What You Fear." *Psychology Today*, Oct 1986 v20 p46(5).

Melzack, Ronald. *The Puzzle of Pain*. New York: Basic Books, 1973.

Melzack, Ronald, and Wall, P.D., The Challenge of Pain, 1982.

Melzack, Ronald, and Wall, P.D. "Pain Mechanisms: A New Theory." *Science*, 150(1965):971-979.

Melzack, Ronald, "The Tragedy of Needless Pain," *Scientific American*, February 1990.

Miller, T.W. *Chronic Pain*, 2 vols., 1990.

Modeland, Vern. "Modern Anesthesia: Going Under Safely." *FDA Consumer*, Dec-Jan 1989 v23 n10 p13(5).

Moyers, Bill. *Healing and The Mind*. New York: Doubleday, 1993.

Olshan, N.H. *Power Over Pain Without Drugs*. New York: Beaufort Books, 1983.

Ornstein, Robert, and Sobel, David. *The Healing Brain: Breakthrough Discoveries About How the Brain Keeps Us Healthy*. New York: Simon & Schuster, 1988.

Ornstein, Robert, and Sobel, David. *Healthy Pleasures*. Reading, MA: Addison-Wesley, 1990.

Oyle, Irving. *The Healing Mind*. New York: Pocket Books, 1975.

Padus, Emrika (ed.). *The Complete Guide to Your Emotions and Your Health*. Emmaus, PA: Rodale Press, 1992.

Papper, Emanuel M. "Anesthesiology Comes of Age." *JAMA, The Journal of the American Medical Association*, Sept 1, 1989 v262 n9 p1225(3)

Pelletier, Kenneth R. *Holistic Medicine: From Stress to Optimum Health*. Magnolia, MA: Peter Smith, 1984.

Pelletier, Kenneth R. *Mind as Healer, Mind as Slayer* (Revised ed.). New York: Delacorte, 1992.

Peterson, Christopher, and Bossio, Lisa M. *Health and Optimism*. New York: Macmillan, 1991.

Pilisuk, Marc, and Parks, Susan H. *The Healing Web: Social Networks and Human Survival*. Hanover, NH: University Press of New England, 1986.

Policoff, Stephen Phillip. "The Mind/Body Link." *Ladies Home Journal*, Oct 1990 v107 n10 p126(4).

Ress, Alan M., and Hoffman, Catherine. *Consumer Health Information Source Book* (3rd ed.). Phoenix: Oryx Press, 1990.

Richardson, A. *Mental Imagery*. New York: Springer, 1969.

Rossi, Ernest L. *The Psychobiology of Mind-Body Healing*. New York: W.W. Norton, 1986.

Rossi, Ernest L., and Cheek, David. *Mind-Body Therapy: Methods of Ideodynamic Healing in Hypnosis*. New York: W.W. Norton, 1988.

Rossman, Martin L. *Healing Yourself: A Step-by-Step Program for Better Health Through Imagery*. New York: Walker, 1987.

Samuels, Michael. *Healing with the Mind's Eye*. New York: Random House, 1992.

Sebel, Peter; Bonke, Benno; Winograd, Eugene (eds.). *Memory and Awareness in Anesthesia*. Englewood Cliffs, NJ: PTR Prentice-Hall, 1993.

Selye, Hans. *The Stress of Life* (2nd ed.). New York: McGraw-Hill, 1978.

Shealy, C. Norman. *The Pain Game*. Berkeley: Celestial Arts, 1976.

Sheikh, A.A. (ed.) *Imagination and Healing*. Farmingdale, NY: Baywood, 1984.

Siegel, Bernie. *How To Live Between Office Visits*. New York: Harper-Collins, 1993.

Siegel, Bernie. *Love, Medicine and Miracles*. New York: Harper & Row, 1986.

Siegel, Bernie. *Peace, Love, and Healing*. New York: Harper & Row, 1989.

Simonton, O. Carl; Matthews-Simonton; and Creighton, James. *Getting Well Again*. New York: Bantam Books, 1980.

Sobel, Davis S. (ed.). *Ways of Health: Holistic Approaches in Ancient and Contemporary Medicine*. New York: Harcourt Brace Jovanovich, 1979.

Spiegel, David. *Living Beyond Limits*. New York: New York Times Books, 1993.

Stacy, Charles B.; Kaplan, Andrew S.; and Williams, Gray. *The Fight Against Pain*. Yonkers, NY: Consumer Reports Books, 1992.

Stocker-Ferguson, Sharon. "Get a Dose of Medicinal Videos. (Mental Imagery Therapy)." *Prevention*, Dec 1990 v42 n12 p60(8).

Strasburg, Kate; Saper, Rob; Joss, Jennifer and Lerner, Michael. *The Quest for Wholeness: An Annotated Bibliography in Patient-Centered Medicine*. Bolinas, CA: Commonweal, 1991.

Stutz, David, and Feder, Bernard. *The Savvy Patient: How to Be an Active Participant in Your Medical Care*. Yonkers, NY: Consumer Reports Books, 1990.

Turk, D.C.; Meichenbaum, D.; and Genest, M. *Pain and Behavioral Medicine: A Cognitive-Behavioral Perspective*. New York: Guilford Press, 1983.

Ulene, Art. *Feeling Fine*. Los Angeles: J.P. Tarcher, 1977.

Wallnofer, Heinrich, and von Rottauscher, Anna. *Chinese Folk Medicine*. New York: Signet, 1972.

Warfield, C.A. (ed.). *Manual of Pain Management*, 1990.

Williams, Gurney, III. "Pain! Treating it and Defeating it." *American Health: Fitness of Body and Mind*, Nov 1991 v10 n9 p45(3).

# Index

# About the Authors

## MONICA WINEFRYDE FURLONG, M.D.

British-born doctor Monica Furlong graduated from the School of Medicine of the University of Leeds in England and completed her internship and residency in anesthesiology at Mt. Sinai Hospital in New York. Dr. Furlong is presently an attending anesthesiologist at Beth Israel Medical Center North (formerly Doctors Hospital) in New York City. She is a Diplomate of the American Board of Anesthesiology.

Dr. Furlong has conducted two research studies on awareness under general anesthesia. Her studies demonstrated the benefits of giving audio taped suggestions to patients undergoing surgery. Dr. Furlong presented the results of her studies at medical conferences in Glasgow, New York, and Atlanta.

Dr. Furlong has also lectured on awareness and anesthesia in England, Israel and in the United States. A firm believer in awareness under anesthesia, Dr. Furlong stresses the importance of emotional support both before and during surgery. In addition, she has called for a greater level of sensitivity by operating room personnel to patient awareness.

## ELLIOT T. ESSMAN

New York native Elliot Essman is a prolific writer, editor and publisher. Originally a legal journalist, Mr. Essman has written several non-fiction books, among them *Life in the USA: A Complete Guide for Immigrants and Americans* and *Building Yourself: Putting Success Together One Piece at a Time*. Mr. Essman's book and film reviews have appeared in numerous publications. He writes a regular newspaper column entitled "People in Love." An active public speaker, Mr. Essman has lectured on love, human relationships, and self developmental topics in the United States, Canada, and several countries in Europe.

Mr. Essman's novel, *A Fool Like Me*, and his work of poetry, *1968*, will both be published in 1994.

# Control Over Your Surgical and Postsurgical Pain

The mission and motive of this book is to give you, the surgical patient, maximum control over your own anesthesia and pain control experience. This book is filled with information and techniques to help you feel less pain and go home from the hospital sooner after your surgery.

If you would like to know more about new advances in mind/body healing and pain control, or if you would like information on how to order cassette tapes for use before, during or after your surgery, please send us your name and address. Our address is:

Autonomy Publishing Corporation
501 East 87th Street, Suite 15B
New York, NY 10128

Of course — any questions and comments about this book are welcome.